Health Commu

Accession no.
36220211

Health Communication

A Media and Cultural Studies Approach

Belinda Lewis
Monash University, Australia

Jeff Lewis
RMIT University, Australia

LIS LIBRARY

Date	Fund
23/03/16	xp-Shr

Order No
2718443

University of Chester

 macmillan
education   palgrave

© Belinda Lewis and Jeff Lewis 2015

All rights reserved. No reproduction, copy or transmission of this publication may be made without written permission.

No portion of this publication may be reproduced, copied or transmitted save with written permission or in accordance with the provisions of the Copyright, Designs and Patents Act 1988, or under the terms of any licence permitting limited copying issued by the Copyright Licensing Agency, Saffron House, 6–10 Kirby Street, London EC1N 8TS.

Any person who does any unauthorized act in relation to this publication may be liable to criminal prosecution and civil claims for damages.

The authors have asserted their rights to be identified as the authors of this work in accordance with the Copyright, Designs and Patents Act 1988.

First published 2015 by
PALGRAVE

Palgrave in the UK is an imprint of Macmillan Publishers Limited, registered in England, company number 785998, of 4 Crinan Street, London N1 9XW.

Palgrave Macmillan in the US is a division of St Martin's Press LLC, 175 Fifth Avenue, New York, NY 10010.

Palgrave is a global imprint of the above companies and is represented throughout the world.

Palgrave® and Macmillan® are registered trademarks in the United States, the United Kingdom, Europe and other countries.

ISBN 978–0–230–29832–3

This book is printed on paper suitable for recycling and made from fully managed and sustained forest sources. Logging, pulping and manufacturing processes are expected to conform to the environmental regulations of the country of origin.

A catalogue record for this book is available from the British Library.

A catalog record for this book is available from the Library of Congress.

Printed in China

Contents

List of Illustrations

Figures

Tables

Plates

Boxes

Acknowledgements

The authors would like to acknowledge and thank the following people for use of their materials: Margaret Whitehead for Figure 1.1 The Main Determinants of Health: An Ecological Model; Act-Belong-Commit for Figure 5.1; Summer Foundation Ambassador Michelle Newland for Plate 7.1; Dr Patricia Fagan and Heather Roberston, Queensland Health, for their case study of Kasa Por Yarn, Chapter 8; Kasa Por Yarn acknowledges the Torres Strait Island and NPA community members who contributed to and supported KPY; Actors in Kasa Por Yarn Series 1, Rhian Phineasa, Danny Bani and Talei Elu, for Plate 8.1 and Heather Robertson as the photographer; Zed books for Figure 9.1 Integrated Strategy Plan Example; Summer Foundation for Figure 10.2 and the media release used as the basis for Figure 10.4; Summer Foundation Ambassador Kirrily Hayward for Plate 10.1 and Fred Kroh as the photographer.

The authors would also like to acknowledge the support of Monash and RMIT universities, and the Australian Research Council. Thanks also to the following people who have provided feedback and assistance – Amberlee Laws, Arvind Singhal, Ben Smith, Di Winkler, Frances Doran, Heather Robertson, Helen Hall, Kate Carmichael, Kirsten Millman, Kirsty Best, Louise Farnworth, Meagan Down, Paul James, Rob Donovan, Sharyn Crawford and Tsharni Zazryn.

Thanks to Kate Llewellyn and others in the Palgrave team who have supported this project over a long period. We also thank each of the four academic reviewers for their comments and suggestions.

We express particular appreciation to Sian Lewis for her outstanding contribution to the development, writing and editing of this book. Your intelligent and thoughtful perspectives were essential to every part of this project. Thanks also to Jay Lewis whose constant support and encouragement have been invaluable. Thank you to Meg, Arthur, Geraldine, Anne-Marie, George, Frances, Ian, Jeremy and Gezza, the wild-eyed kelpie, our parents and all members of the family. Your friendship and love have carried us through.

Introduction

This book is about communicating for health and social change. It is focused on working with media, culture and communities to bring about changes to the conditions of people's lives, to improve their opportunities for health and contribute to a more equitable and healthful society.

The book brings the perspectives of contemporary media and cultural studies to the field of health communication. It outlines and explains the contribution that media and cultural studies has to offer students, scholars and practitioners of health communication in the context of public health and health promotion practice.

Moving beyond the focus on conventional approaches, this book elucidates the central role of media and culture in health communication. It explores the complex and dynamic world of the mass media and interactive, digital media environments to offer new insights into the challenges and opportunities for communicating about health. Through its thematic approach, the book lays out key theories and critical debates in media and cultural studies and, using a diverse range of practical case studies, illustrates how these may usefully inform health communication scholarship and practice.

Aims of this book

In this book, we offer an introduction to media and cultural studies perspectives. We show how their insights offer ways of understanding how 'health' is being communicated in contemporary contexts – not just in terms of information and education, but as communities and cultures through a diverse range of sources, influences and actions. We use this approach to open up discussions about the place of the media within the meanings and practices of people's everyday lives.

Cultural studies provides a sophisticated approach to understanding the complex dynamics of culture and social change – and the ways this is mediated in contemporary societies. Rather than thinking of cultural studies as an 'alternative' approach, we see it as a complement to other approaches already being used in health communication. Furthermore, by using a media and cultural studies approach as a lens to examine how we communicate in our health communication interventions, we have new tools to help explain their success and failures in addressing complex public health issues. These new perspectives can help us to explore the opportunities and challenges of working with media to generate social change – and to build on the strengths of existing strategies.

We hope that the discussions in this book will offer new insights and an original contribution to theory and practice in health communication. In the

I

process of being read, studied and critiqued by students, researchers and practitioners, we hope it will forge new and innovative links between the academic disciplines of health communication and media and cultural studies.

Structure of the book

Part I of the book explores culture, communication and health and introduces a cultural studies approach. We examine the structure and dynamics of the mediasphere and the various roles of the media. Contemporary theories and models for understanding production, representation, audiences and meaning-making are introduced. We illustrate these ideas through a diverse array of practical case studies and contemporary issues. Part II presents a range of practical approaches for health communication: social marketing, participatory communication, community media-making, entertainment-education, community activism and public health advocacy. Each chapter is focused on a different approach, with strategies and skills explained using practical examples and insights from experienced practitioners.

We have structured this book so that the theoretical discussions in the earlier chapters of the book (Part I) are further developed through application and discussion in relation to a range of health communication approaches (Part II). Each approach is discussed in a separate chapter, covering

- definitions, models and underpinning theory;
- strengths and limitations in relation to health promotion;
- practical case studies;
- application of new digital technologies and the Internet;
- frameworks for integrating this approach into multi-strategy health promotion.

PART I

Understanding Media and Culture in Health Communication

Media, Culture and Communication in Health Promotion

Introduction

This chapter provides an introduction to contemporary health communication and health promotion. Beginning with the controversial *Grim Reaper* HIV/AIDS campaign in Australia, we explore the limitations of earlier approaches to health communication and their evolution towards the socio-ecological approach that underpins contemporary health promotion.

This chapter demonstrates the political nature of contemporary health communication. We argue that the media is implicated in all health promotion strategies. This means that all people working in public health and health promotion need new ways of understanding the role of the media and the interactions between media, culture, experts and communities.

We introduce media and cultural studies as a framework for understanding the complex dynamics of the media, its relationship with culture and its role in health promotion. We argue that participatory approaches to health communication are essential if we are to facilitate opportunities for communities themselves to *enable, mediate* and *advocate* for health and social change.

Always use condoms, always!

In Australia, the first death from AIDS occurred in 1983. By 1987, HIV/AIDS was recognised as a serious disease causing death and debilitating illness for significant numbers of people, and the Australian government launched its first mass media campaign to raise public awareness about the disease. The first and most controversial TV advertisement depicted the *Grim Reaper*, a hooded, decomposing and faceless creature, holding up a scythe, and rolling a ten-pin bowling ball down an alley – knocking down horrified men, women and child 'pins' which represented AIDS victims. The final grim voiceover warned, 'Always use condoms, always!'

Criticised for its gruesome imagery, scare tactics and blunt message, the fear campaign dramatically raised anxieties in the population at large (those least at risk), but it barely affected the behaviour amongst people in communities most at risk (homosexual men and IV drug users). Before long, epidemiologists confirmed that the virus had emerged through the gay community. Panic amongst the general population died down, along with what had turned out to be only small, short-term increases in their condom use. Instead of leading to an informed and responsible public prepared to use condoms during sex, the campaign was far more effective at identifying gay men as the source of the 'killer epidemic' resulting in stigmatisation, discrimination, bullying, vilification and violence against gay men.

The *Grim Reaper* campaign not only failed to change sexual behaviour amongst the audience it most needed to reach, but it also generated outrage amongst the gay community. What followed was one of the most effective examples of grass-roots communication about health over that decade. As mainstream media organisations became increasingly reluctant to cover what was perceived to be a 'gay disease', media activism by and for people with HIV/AIDS filled the gap, helping to create an alternative public sphere for the exchange of experiences, knowledge and opinions. In contrast to the US$3 million broadcast advertising provided by government medical authorities, new forms of narrowcast communication emerged. Information about reducing risks, gay-friendly health services and testing and treatment for HIV/AIDS began circulating through networks of gay communities in Sydney via community radio stations and alternative press, gay bars and venues and sex worker collectives.

Instead of passively accepting scrutiny and blame, gay communities were mobilising: gay and bisexual men, their partners and supporters rallied together to offer alternative portrayals of the human suffering and sadness of living and dying with HIV/AIDS and the impacts on loved ones and families. Strident activists and high-profile gay public figures featured in news reports, talk shows and a host of public gatherings, speaking articulately and with compassion about the need for non-discriminatory, affordable and accessible health care and prevention strategies for all members of Gay, Lesbian, Bisexual, Transgender, Intersex (LGBTI) and sex worker communities. Politicians, public health authorities and other decision-makers responded.

Contemporaneous with similar activities in New York, San Francisco and London, even Hollywood got on board in 1993, releasing *Philadelphia*, one of the first films to present a sympathetic portrayal of AIDS, homosexuality and the impact of homophobia. This was followed by a plethora of other films, documentaries, TV programmes, biographies and novels – with many featuring and/or written by people with HIV/AIDS, their lovers, family and friends. These mediated discourses and narratives contributed to a gradual shift in public perceptions and understanding about HIV/AIDS. Rather than seeing the disease as retribution for the excesses of non-mainstream sexual orientations, relationships and lifestyles, the public became increasingly aware that HIV/AIDS was a sexually transmitted infection – an everyday risk as part of contemporary relationships and cultural life. Diverse media representations of gay and bisexual relationships helped to fortify this cultural transformation.

Health promotion and health communication

The failings of the *Grim Reaper* media campaign reflect the limitations of earlier approaches to health communication and health promotion. These earlier approaches demonstrate a limited understanding of the media and the interactions between media, culture, experts and publics (communities). So, let's now have a closer look at what is meant by health communication and health promotion.

Health promotion is the process of enabling people to increase control over their health as well as the factors that influence their health. It involves various, planned combinations of educational, political, regulatory and organisational supports for actions and conditions of living conducive to the health of individuals, groups and communities (World Health Organization 2009).

Communication is fundamental to every aspect of health promotion. Traditionally, the field of health communication has been informed by psychology, social marketing and early theories of mass communication. The focus has been on providing information, education and health messages to influence people's attitudes, beliefs and behaviours as well as the factors that influence their behaviour choices. However, more recent scholarship and practice has seen health communication evolve from its earlier roots in an individualised, medical model of health towards the socio-ecological approach that underpins contemporary health promotion.

As Wilkinson and Marmot (2003) have argued, 'while medical care can prolong survival, more important for the health of the population as a whole are the social and economic conditions that actually make people ill and need of medical care' (p.7). The ecological approach provides a framework for understanding and addressing the factors that influence people's health. Within this approach, health communication has expanded its earlier focus on provision of health information to embrace new forms of 'communication for health' in which health practitioners work in partnership 'with' communities rather than 'on' them. It involves facilitating opportunities for people's everyday participation in social dialogue and fostering the supportive environments needed for social change to take place. Syme (2004: 3) explains this shift when he says,

[w]e rarely identify and intervene on those forces in the community that cause the problem in the first place ... If we can move away from a singular focus on diseases and risk factors and begin to think about community and social forces, we can also relate to the community in a more meaningful way.

Various models are used to explain the ecological approach, but their common feature is a focus on the multiple levels of influence on people's health. The

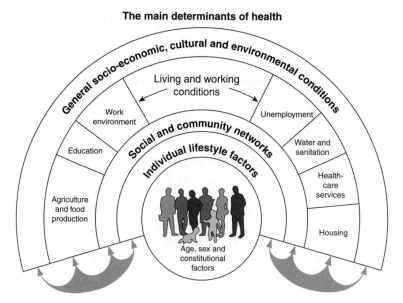

Figure 1.1   The main determinants of health: An ecological model

Source: Dahlgren and Whitehead (1993: 11)

model developed by Dahlgren and Whitehead (1993) describes these influences as interdependent layers that interact with, and influence, each other (see Figure 1.1). Based on the extensive body of evidence about the determinants of health, the model illustrates the fundamental conditions and resources that are prerequisites for health. It begins with individuals at the core, moving out to the wider socio-economic, cultural and environmental factors that influence health for individuals, communities and whole societies.

So, within this context, health communication is gradually extending its traditional focus on creating change primarily at the level of individuals to a more ecological approach in which communication is a means of facilitating change within groups and communities (strengthening social supports and cultural life), living and working conditions (policies and practices in government and organisations) and societal structures (laws and regulations, economic and taxation policies to bring about more equitable access to resources and services, and political action at national and international levels).

Also underpinned by the ecological approach, the Ottawa Charter for Health Promotion (WHO 1986) outlines five 'action areas' for health promotion intervention: reorient health services, develop personal skills, strengthen community action, create supportive environments and build healthy public policy. In each of these areas, effective communication is central to the process of generating change. This means that public health researchers and health promotion practitioners need a range of communication strategies and skills in order to work with a wide range of stakeholders, including other sectors, governments, local authorities, industries, non-government and voluntary organisations, community groups and the media (WHO 1986: 2). These may include:

- Contributing to public debates about priority health problems and risks to health; causes of health problems; and solutions to health problems and strategies for promoting health.
- Advocating for systemic political change to address the underlying causes of health problems.
- Mediating between the perspectives of different, and often competing, interests in society about responsibility for health problems and strategies for change.
- Enabling and empowering community members to voice their experiences and perspectives and take an active role in public decision-making (WHO 1986).

The World Health Organization repeatedly emphasises that 'at the heart of this process is the empowerment of communities, their ownership and control of their own endeavours and destinies' (1986: 3). Accordingly, it is essential to develop health communication strategies with a focus on social justice, community empowerment and capacity-building in order to help communities access the skills, confidence and resources that people need to take an active role in communicating for health.

Dutta (2011) argues that the effectiveness of health communication should be assessed by its capacity to facilitate 'participation' in social change. For Dutta, the term 'communication for social change' refers to an emerging field of communication focused on challenging and transforming global, national and local structures of power that create and sustain inequalities and oppressive conditions for poor and/or marginalised communities. This approach involves creating points of access for marginalised groups themselves to strategically participate in communicative practices in ways that transform the conditions of their everyday lives. Central to this work are processes of empowerment through:

- engagement in dialogue
- consciousness-raising
- sharing information
- forming networks and collectives
- community mobilising and advocacy.

This process involves creating greater opportunities for education, literacy and access to the Internet and digital communication technologies. It also includes facilitating new connections between local and global networks of people interested in bringing about social transformation (Curry Jansen et al. 2011).

As we explore throughout this book, participatory approaches to health communication are essential if we are to facilitate opportunities for communities themselves to *enable, mediate* and *advocate* for health and social change.

These approaches are pivotal if people are to gain more control over the decisions and resources that affect their lives and health (Dutta 2011). The media and cultural studies approach that we are adopting in this book provides a framework for understanding how contemporary health communication functions within the ecological model of health.

Contemporary health communication is political

Our discussions this far demonstrate the political nature of contemporary health communication. Health is an unequally distributed resource. There are many contested claims over the best ways to address the wider social and economic structural causes of illness, injury and inequalities in health (WHO 2008). These debates are influenced by the priorities and values of decision-makers in organisations and governments, and the powerful interest groups who seek to influence these decision-makers.

Clearly then, health is also about power and control. Those with greater access to power, resources and the media have greater capacity to set the agenda, to identify health 'problems' and to influence public discussion and debate about appropriate solutions. These politics influence the public agenda around health: that is, which issues receive attention and which are excluded, whose voices are represented and whose are marginalised. Thus, public decision-making about health-related issues and distribution of resources is strongly shaped by the values, ideological and economic interests of those with greatest access to these communicative spaces – powerful individuals, big corporations, professional and industry lobby groups, governments and transnational organisations. To this extent, health is an issue with many political dimensions at the global and local level. Communicating about health, therefore, is always political (Dutta 2011; Tulloch & Lupton 1997).

Within the contemporary media, public health itself is a zone of intense struggle and contestation. But within this context, new opportunities and challenges for health promotion are being created. As we will explore throughout this book, people are producing, sharing and exchanging information and ideas about health in a multitude of ways. Communities are taking action to change the factors that influence their opportunities for healthy lives by using new modes of communication to form coalitions and alliances and engage in strategies to influence decision-makers in communities, corporations and governments.

We can relate this to the HIV/AIDS *Grim Reaper* case study. By organising for their social and legal rights, LGBTI and sex worker communities successfully mobilised improved resources for sexual health education, health clinics, outreach programmes and advocacy. They formed activist groups, such as ACT-UP (AIDS Coalition to Unleash Power), and advocacy organisations, such as AIDS Councils, that have continued working for decades to address misconceptions about HIV/AIDS, diverse sexualities and sex workers and also to generate political action for longer term change (Laverack

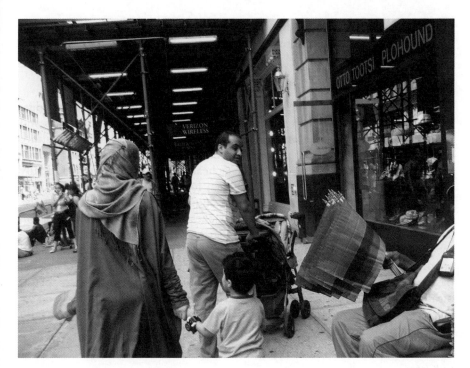

Plate 1.1   Supporters attending Gay Pride March

Source: Belinda Lewis

2013). As we will discuss in chapters 6, 7, 8 and 9, advocacy organisations and community groups, such as these, provide important spaces for 'active citizenship' and a collective political presence aimed at overcoming oppression, stigma, discrimination and disconnection. They also offer diverse opportunities for health promotion, entertainment and social support within the wider community.

The role of media and culture

In almost all health promotion strategies, the media is implicated – either directly or indirectly. Some strategies are focused directly on the media, such as public health information and social marketing campaigns. In others, the media is fundamental to their effectiveness, including community development, community mobilising, and advocacy for policy change and legislative reform. Health promotion practitioners engage proactively with the media, and they also respond to media news coverage and entertainment content that has implications for health. Increasingly, health promotion experts are also being called upon to engage in public debates about regulation of media content and restrictions on advertising that may undermine health (Chapman 2007). Accordingly, all people working in public health, health promotion and health communication need a sound understanding of the role of the media and culture in health promotion.

Power and participation

While health communication has traditionally privileged 'expert' knowledge, recent approaches place greater emphasis on people's own understandings and personal experience, commonsense knowledge and the centrality of culture (Zoller & Dutta 2008). The power and control that medical and health professionals have traditionally wielded over health communication is gradually being challenged through approaches which foster community empowerment and capacity-building. In practice, health communication is gradually evolving from expert-driven, top-down approaches using information, education and social marketing to include more participatory approaches. These are focused around entertainment, community media, community activism and advocacy for healthy public policy. Audiences are less likely to be considered passive 'receivers' of health communication but rather active participants in meaning-making and 'media-making'. It is this context which is driving an increasing interest in understanding the role of media and culture in health communication.

Culture

Culture is central to health communication. Most health communication research and practice has been underpinned by fairly limited concepts of culture as referring to the particular shared beliefs and practices of specific ethnic, religious and marginalised groups. These understandings are then used to assist practitioners and researchers to better engage with various cultural groups, to overcome culture as a 'barrier' to change and to tailor health messages and actions accordingly (Dutta 2008; Corcoran 2007). Emerging approaches to more 'culture-centred' health communication present an alternative perspective in which culture, rather than being seen as a barrier, is instead *central* to effective health communication. Culture-centred approaches provide 'an avenue for opening up the dominant framework for health communication to communities and contexts that have so far been ignored, rendered silent and treated simply as subjects of health communication interventions' (Dutta 2008: 14).

Cultural studies offers new ways of understanding culture in the context of health communication by interrogating what culture is and how it is shared. Culture is a crucial concept for understanding the ways in which we interact with each other, the media and significant fields of knowledge and information. In an increasingly complex, globalising world, social groups and their cultures are understood as being dynamic, overlapping and perpetually changing. This understanding of culture is pivotal if we are to engage with communities in meaningful ways to negotiate change. Culture is the central platform for these negotiations: it is not an impediment, but a space in which we might explore opportunities. Culture is constantly 'in the making' and the media has a central place in the processes by which culture is created and shared, contested and transformed.

Media and cultural studies

To date, the disciplines of health promotion and public health have only barely engaged with the disciplines of media and cultural studies (Seale 2004, 2002). This engagement has been mostly in terms of critical analysis of media content and the evaluation of the effectiveness of mass communication campaigns (Germov & Freij 2009; Abroms & Maibach 2008). Within public health and health promotion, there have been few attempts to genuinely examine the complex dynamics of the media environment and its relationship with culture and social change.

Health promotion policy and practice can be advanced by new understandings of the role of the media in shaping (and being shaped by) community attitudes and practices. As we explain in Chapter 2 (see Figure 2.1, p.21), the Cultural Model of Media proposes that this dynamic takes place between four levels within the 'mediasphere' (Lewis 2002; Hartley 1996), including texts, audiences, media-makers and the cultural-governance contexts in which they operate. Circulating within the mediasphere is a complex and interactive web of messages and meanings about health. Some are driven by public health experts, health professionals and health promotion practitioners. Others reflect dominant discourses on health underpinned by the ideologies of powerful social groups and commercial vested interests. Furthermore, as people communicate with each other as part of everyday life, a diverse array of stories, images, texts and meanings about health are continually being created through entertainment and popular culture.

Cultural studies approaches to health communication acknowledge that media audiences are not passive receivers of messages, but are actively engaged in the production and adaption of meanings (Lewis 2008). Inevitably, people generate multiple meanings from these media texts depending on their own personal experiences, significant social groups, knowledge systems, cultural practices and beliefs. They interact with media texts and their respective cultures in order to make sense of their lives and the world around them. A cultural approach explores the ways in which media-makers and audiences interact around media to actively produce meanings, attitudes and values. Within this approach, health communication is not assumed to be a top-down, expert-led process of developing the 'right messages' to change the beliefs and practices of individuals. Instead, it is conceived as a process of exchange in which meanings are constantly being produced, contested and reproduced by audiences. That is, audiences themselves are actively engaged in meaning-making and also the process of media-making. People themselves become agents of change through their engagement with – and influence on – various media and new modes of communication (see Chapter 2).

Furthermore, new digital technologies and the convergence of the media industries are radically changing the ways in which the media function. This dynamic and interactive media environment is altering media production, distribution and consumption. There are now many forms of media other than corporate mass media that influence people's attitudes and values. A plethora of media-making is also happening at the community level using digital technologies and the Internet for social networking and community-building, development, community mobilising, advocacy and activism (Ricketts 2012; Dutta 2011; Pullen & Cooper 2010). A media and cultural studies approach examines the wider factors that influence production of media texts and identifies opportunities for facilitating the engagement of audiences themselves in media-making at the professional and community level. This approach also provides a framework for engaging with emerging critical debates about health communication within rapidly changing media environments and the practical implications for health professionals and the public.

Cultural studies offers new ways of understanding the relationship between media, culture and communication, and it helps to explain the successes and failures of communication campaigns to address complex public health issues. By moving beyond traditional, linear, top-down models of media influence, and expanding the parameters for understanding new media environments, it is possible to open up innovative opportunities for health promotion policy and practice. A media and cultural studies approach explores the opportunities and challenges of utilising media to generate social change and to build on the strengths of existing approaches.

Bridging the disciplinary divide

Over the past decade, as we have noted above, the media itself has been rapidly evolving in both industrialised and developing country contexts. The rise of interactive, mobile, digital communication technologies and social media has enabled exponential growth in user-generated content. Along with convergence of media forms and changes to the production of news, this increasingly global and more participatory environment is contributing to a very dynamic media landscape. Within media and cultural studies, new theories and lively critical debates continue to emerge around the possibilities, challenges and socio-cultural implications of these emerging media forms (Lewis, 2005).

While health promotion and public health practitioners seek to mobilise the media in their work, they often find they are dealing with new forms of communication that are not yet fully understood and the impact of which they cannot fully control. Not surprisingly then, most health communication literature has continued the traditional focus on the following:

1. Health information, education and behaviour change focused communication, delivering messages to the public through mass media campaigns and various digital technologies.
2. Sociology of media and health, including patterns of media use and critical analysis of media representations.

3. Psychology-based studies evaluating the 'effects' of various media on different audience groups.

In recent years, however, public health researchers and practitioners have expressed a growing interest in developing a deeper understanding of the role of media and culture in relation to public health. Key health communication scholars have called for a 'revision of existing models of health communication and construction of alternate models of practice' and propose approaches that we 'open up the spaces of health communication to the voices of cultural communities' (Zoller & Dutta 2008). Researchers and practitioners have also been encouraged to engage more actively with the disciplines of media and cultural studies as a 'framework for understanding the complex place that media can have in people's lives' (Seale 2002). This will be the focus of the next chapter.

References

Abroms, L. and Maibach, E. 2008, 'The effectiveness of mass communication to change public behaviour', *Annual Reviews of Public Health*, 29: 219–234.

Chapman, S. 2007, *Public Health Advocacy and Tobacco Control: Making Smoking History*, Blackwell, Oxford.

Corcoran, N. 2007, *Communicating Health: Strategies for Health Promotion*, Sage, London.

Curry Jansen, S., Pooley, J. and Taub-Pervizpour, L. 2011, *Media and Social Justice*, Palgrave Macmillan, New York.

Dahlgren, G. and Whitehead, M. 1993, Tackling inequalities in health: What can we learn from what has been tried? Working paper prepared for the King's Fund International Seminar on Tackling Inequalities in Health, September 1993, Ditchley Park, Oxfordshire. London, King's Fund, accessible in: Dahlgren, G. and Whitehead, M. 2007, *European Strategies for Tackling Social Inequities in Health: Levelling up Part 2*. Copenhagen: WHO Regional office for Europe. Accessed 6 May 2014 http://www.euro.who.int/__data/assets/pdf_file/0018/103824/E89384.pdf.

Dutta, M. 2008, *Communicating Health: A Culture-Centered Approach*, Polity, London.

Dutta, M. 2011, *Communicating Social Change: Structure, Culture, and Agency*, Routledge, New York.

Germov, J. and Freij, M. 2009, 'Media and health', in J. Germov (ed.) *Second Opinion: An Introduction to Health Sociology*, 4th Edition, Oxford University Press, Sydney, 347–359.

Hartley, J. 1996, *Popular Reality: Journalism, Modernity, Popular Culture*, Arnold, London.

Laverack, G. 2013, *Health Activism: Foundations and Strategies*, Sage, London.

Lewis, J. 2002, *Cultural Studies*, Sage, London.

Lewis, J. 2005, *Language Wars: The Role of Media and Culture in Global Terror and Political Violence*, Pluto Books, London.

Lewis, J. 2008, *Cultural Studies*, 2nd Edition, London, Sage.

Pullen, C. and Cooper, M. (eds.) 2010, *LGBT Identity and Online New Media*, Routledge, New York.

Ricketts, A. 2012, *The Activists Handbook: A Step-By-Step Guide to Participatory Democracy*, Zed Books, London.

Seale, C. 2002, *Media and Health*, Sage, London.

Seale, C. 2004, *Health and the Media*, Blackwell, Oxford.

Syme, L. 2004, 'Social determinants of health: The community as an empowered partner', *Preventing Chronic Disease*, 1 (1): 1–5.

Tulloch, J. and Lupton, D. 1997, *Television, AIDS and Risk: A Cultural Studies Approach to Health Communication*, Allen & Unwin, St Leonards.

Wilkinson, R. and Marmot, M. (eds) 2003, *Social Determinants of Health: The Solid Facts*, 2nd Edition, World Health Organization, Denmark. Accessed 6 May 2014 www.euro.who.int/__data/assets/pdf_file/0005/98438/e81384.pdf.

World Health Organization 1986, Ottawa charter for health promotion, in WHO 2009, *Milestones in Health Promotion: Statements from Global Conferences*, WHO/NMH/CHP/09.01, 1–5. Accessed 6 May 2014 http://www.who.int/healthpromotion/Milestones_Health_Promotion_05022010.pdf.

World Health Organization 2008, *Closing the Gap in a Generation: Health Equity through Action on the Social Determinants of Health. Final Report of the Commission on Social Determinants of Health*. World Health Organization, Geneva. Accessed 6 May 2014 http://www.who.int/social_determinants/thecommission/finalreport/en/index.html.

World Health Organization 2009, *Health Promotion*. Accessed 6 May 2014 http://www.who.int/topics/health_promotion/en/.

Zoller, H. and Dutta, M. 2008, *Emerging Perspectives in Health Communication: Meaning, Culture and Power*, Routledge, New York.

Understanding the Media

2

Chapter overview

This chapter provides an introduction to the role of the media and culture in contemporary society. We trace the origins of the modern media from its early beginnings as a source of information to the integral role that media now occupy in almost every aspect of modern societies. The chapter explores the strengths and limitations of different theoretical approaches to understanding the role of the media in health promotion and public health communication. We argue that media are diverse and complex, and we challenge older, linear models of media influence. We introduce the cultural model of the media using examples of the 2011 royal wedding and the performance art of feminist punk-band Pussy Riot. We argue that health professionals need to engage with all forms of media, and particularly interactive and community media, that engage community members as active participants in shaping better health outcomes.

Introduction to the role of media: Information, economy and pleasure

The origins of the modern media

As it is generally understood, the media is the apparatus that allows members of a mass society to share information, ideas, images, stories, emotions, beliefs and various modes of entertainment. The media, in this sense, are not simply communication service providers, but are an integral part of the way members of modern societies talk to one another and imagine their social bonds and sense of belonging. Thus, the media are fundamentally engaged in the ways in which we conceive of ourselves, each other and our world.

Cultural studies scholar, Benedict Anderson (2006), argues that the emergence of the first mass media technology, the printing press, was critical to the formation of the modern nation. Mass printing and literacy, Anderson claims, are a prerequisite for effective administration, information-sharing and organisation of large and diverse national populations. Equally, the printing press facilitated the sharing of ideas, political views and stories (narratives) which flesh out a society and its sense of being.

If we consider this claim against all the media that now proliferate in modern societies, we can see that the media are essential to all the knowledge, stories and debates that occur across our public sphere. While we don't know every member of the whole society or community with which we identify, the media provides us with some sense of their presence and proximity. The media tells us about particular kinds of shared language, institutions, knowledge, ideas, laws and stories. And even when we challenge these ideas and perspectives – particularly around moral and political issues – this is an acceptable part of our democratic system. Inscribed into modern democracy is the expectation of some authorised level of dispute and disagreement: a healthy democracy involves the peaceful resolution of these disputes.

The modern, democratic society and its 'public sphere' have themselves been facilitated by the media. Nineteenth-century political philosopher, Thomas Carlyle, described the news media as the 'fourth estate' of modern society. According to Carlyle, the news media and journalism sit with government, education and religion as the foundation of a modern democracy. The public could only make astute electoral decisions, Carlyle believed, if they were well informed and governments were held to account by objective news reporting.

Along with many other media scholars, James Curran (2011) argues that this 'fourth estate' role remains an integral part of the media today. Curran argues that public understanding and political judgements about important issues depend upon mass media's capacity to generate and deliver accurate, balanced and unbiased information to citizens. Within this model, journalism is the pinnacle of the information professions; journalists are the source of all significant social knowledge and the viability of democratic states. In the modern context, Curran argues, citizens are continually distracted from this information by the vast armada of entertainments and fictions that the media also present.

While Curran sees these entertainments as a distraction from the more serious role of the media, it is very clear that story-telling and fiction have always been a part of human culture. Daniel Cohen (2000) argues that mass literacy translated this public taste for sensationalism and scandal into the more general field of journalism and mediation. According to Cohen, these public preferences and pleasures were taken directly into the broadcast and mass print industries that emerged during the 20th century. The modern media and commercial news broadcasting, in particular, have simply extended the 'sensationalism' that characterised earlier forms of information and entertainment (info-tainment).

Entertainment, pleasure and society

The entertainment functions of the media are not simply frivolous; nor are they just a subsidiary of the more 'serious' roles of social organisation, democracy and information sharing. Indeed, while many scholars foreground the fourth estate function of the media, we also need to acknowledge the importance of media as a source of pleasure, and that pleasure itself often has a political, educative and knowledge-building function. We need only consider the fate of Russian feminist punk-band, Pussy Riot, who staged a provocative anti-government performance on the altar of Moscow's Cathedral of Christ the Saviour in 2012. Known for their wild and anarchic lyrics, the band had become famous for opposing the legitimacy of President Vladimir Putin. Three of the women band members were arrested and convicted of 'hooliganism', receiving a two-year prison sentence in an isolated penitentiary.

Like other countries that censor and strictly control the media, Russia exposed its tyrannical and corrupt governmental system through its treatment of the political entertainers. More broadly, however, Pussy Riot are also part of a transnational celebrity culture and its abundant store of images, emotions, information, ideas and stories. And while Pussy Riot and other bands, movie stars and sports stars may use their fame and modes of entertainment to challenge social and political conventions, a number of other celebrities are embedded in a more conservative politics and relatively conventional practices and knowledge systems.

Indeed, a great deal of media – news, entertainment, celebrity – is generated around commerce and profit. Inevitably, mass media spectacles like the 2011 marriage of Prince William and Kate Middleton are part of a media system that consolidates relatively simple commercial principles. As probably the most watched media event in history (Lewis 2013), the royal wedding represented a political confirmation of the global capitalist system. Indeed, unlike the Pussy Riot performance that challenged political authority, the royal wedding was very much entrenched in conservative political perspectives and the global capitalist economic system.

Nearly two billion people were beguiled by the beauty and glamour of the young couple. The pleasure of the spectacle was intensified by the communal sense of hope that is always inscribed in the ritual of nuptial love. It was as though the whole planet were gathering for a moment of uncompromising pleasure: as though all the difficulties, violence and displeasures of the world were dissolved for that one moment of sheer social bliss.

And yet within the rituals and pleasures of the wedding there lurked another and more contentious shadow. Looking more closely at the symbols of this great media event, we might see the imperialism, political infamy and violence that are contingencies of the regal lineage, sovereignty and imperial authority. The Prince's military uniform was not just a random assortment of colours and styles: it represented the violence by which the British imperial crown had come to colonise and oppress millions of people across the globe. This is not simply an historical relic, but resonates with ongoing social privilege – not just as a pinnacle of British society, but as a symbol of Western, developed-world affluence and global power. It is, in this light, difficult to imagine that a royal wedding in Uganda or Paraguay would attract such global attention.

John Frow (2005) has argued, in fact, that mediated celebrity is largely a substitute for older forms of religion and worship. Whether or not this is true, the point remains that celebrity is a key part of the media's social function (see

Turner 2004). Celebrities are a resource for members of a society to engage with their social world and to make sense of themselves, the people around them, and all the issues and experiences by which they live their everyday lives (Turner 2004). Members of a social group relate to celebrities and the mediated stories in which they are situated. They help to personalise mass society and the complex knowledge systems by which the modern democratic state functions. To this end, celebrities and media personalities are both exceptional and highly familiar as they become integrated into people's everyday lives. Whether they are sportspeople, musicians, actors or even politicians, their mediated fame brings celebrities into our homes and minds.

To this end, all the media – news and narrative – are complex and ultimately political. They are both familiar and exceptional, being part of the mass society and world around us, and profoundly personal and embedded in our everyday lives. They are replete with pleasures and dangers, love and violence, hope and despair, truth and untruth. The media, that is, are as complex as we are.

This chapter will explain some of these complexities, particularly in terms of the images, ideas and knowledge systems that are associated with public health. While later chapters will present a more practical guide for using the media for advocacy, activism, community engagement and public health information campaigns, this chapter explains what the media actually 'is'. Because this is so complex, there is a tendency for media and health scholars to simplify the media in order to facilitate practical outcomes. The problem with this approach is that it leads to confusion and excessive claims about what can be achieved through the deployment of media and media facilities. Our aim, therefore, is to explain the media and its underlying complexities in order to understand how best we might develop effective strategies for health enhancement. The only way to do this, we believe, is to scope our strategies in terms of influence and community engagement. As we will argue, the media are neither good nor bad, nor capable of determining specific social effects or individual behavioural changes. The media, rather, involves complex agencies operating within an equally complex cultural ecology. As we will argue in this chapter, the media does not exist as a simple set of tools, industries or technologies; the media are formed through social relationships and meaning-making processes that are always subject to conditions of power, politics, pleasure and displeasure. Those of us who work with media need to begin with this fundamental understanding if we are to achieve the outcomes we seek.

How the media work: A cultural model

The media are not simply a consort of industries, technologies and professionals who deliver perfectly constructed messages to audiences who passively respond and modify their behaviour and beliefs accordingly. This approach to the media, variously called the 'effects' or 'transmission' model, is popular among those marketing, media and health professionals who believe they can determine and control individuals' behaviour and social lives.

In fact, and as we have already illustrated, the media and communications processes are a good deal more complex than this transmission model acknowledges. The media represent a significant cultural agency that is profoundly implicated in the ways in which individuals and social groups understand and experience the world. The media are not All Powerful as the transmission model appears to assume; nor are they capable of determining attitudes and behaviours. However, through their engagement with people and everyday life, the media can influence attitudes, thinking, imagining, emotions and practices, and vice-a-versa.

In a very real sense, we are in the media and the media is in us. As we shall see in the next chapter, this cognitive (thinking and imagining) engagement with the media occurs through the shared space of culture. Culture encompasses all the meanings that a social group has generated through history and which are available for the construction of new texts, meanings and modes of knowledge.

Figure 2.1 (Lewis 2008) gives a sense of how the media work through these key relationships and meaning-making processes.

Each of the triangle points in this diagram (text, producer and audience/users) is engaged in a two-way flow with every other point; texts, producers and audiences/users all interact with one another within an all-encompassing cultural context. Thus, meanings are generated through the flow of these interactions and are never contained within one point. Meanings, and meaning-making, that is, are only possible through the flow of these interactions. While transmission models of communication and the media assume that meanings, and meaning-making created by text producers, are set within a text and then happily accepted and understood as they were intended by the producer, the cultural model sees meaning as much more dynamic and dependent on a complex of interactions. Meaning, in this sense, is always precarious and always in a state of becoming.

Meanings, in fact, like the minds through which they are formed, are never entirely settled or fixed. Meanings are relative to contexts and time, and also to

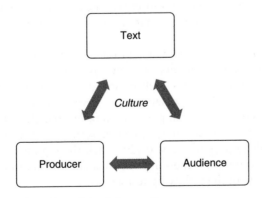

Figure 2.1   The cultural model of the media

Source: Lewis (2008)

the remarkable variability of human individuals and social groups. As we saw in the examples of the British Royal Wedding and Pussy Riot, meanings, in fact, are subject to at least two contending human dispositions: one which would like to fix and stabilise meanings in a durable and unchangeable knowledge system; the other which is always shifting and moving, seeking new possibilities, challenging orthodoxies and power, creating new meanings.

In practical terms, the dynamic nature of meaning-making makes it possible for individuals and groups to change and for the media to assert some degree of influence on these changes. It is also why powerful groups with greater access to media resources are better able to communicate their interests and exert influence on the practices, beliefs and attitudes of others. But it also explains why other social groups are able to challenge these meanings and interests – not only why, for example, tobacco companies were able to encourage smoking practices during the 20th century but also why governments and health advocates have been able to challenge these powerful groups and influence the practices of cigarette smokers.

It is crucially important to keep in mind that social groups come in all sizes and forms – friends, family, ethnic group, workmates, recreational group, religious group, nation, hemisphere, human family. Different groups often share certain values, practices, beliefs, language and so on. However, within these groups, there may also be some very distinctive variations which directly influence the ways in which individuals within the group create meanings and share important knowledge systems. To this end, young people who share a recreational practice, such as clubbing and raves, have distinctive and shared attitudes towards the ways they use certain drugs. These attitudes and practices are formed around a knowledge system that is derived more from their own shared stories and experiences than from scientifically generated public health evidence or society's expert legal institutions. This variability is extremely important because individuals rarely construct meanings in isolation from their significant others: that is the people and social group to which they are most deeply bonded. It is also important because most people living in a mass society, in which they know only a small proportion of the total population, tend to congregate and create their bonds through a number of different social groups – from intimate friendships and communities to much larger 'societies' or 'cultures'.

We will say much more about this in the next chapter, but it is important here to recognise that the media and the processes of meaning-making are entirely bound to this complex web of social relationships and the ways in which individuals in modern societies must navigate a complicated cognitive, emotional and communicational pathway in order to make sense of the world.

The dynamics of meaning-making can be seen in each of the points of the cultural model diagram and the ways in which these points interact with one another. We can summarise these interactions and the cultural context within which they operate in the following terms:

1. Media producers
Media producers include all those people (along with their institutions, communities and processes) who contribute to the production of media texts.

Text producers may be professional and corporate, or non-professional individuals and communities. They include creative people like designers, writers and cinematographers, journalists and information workers, technicians, technocrats, managers, administrators as well as a wide variety of everyday citizens. These individuals, communities and organisations create websites, blogs, photographs, videos, films, songs, pamphlets, clothes and so on. Anything that is designed to create meaning and communicate may be called a media text. Producers draw on the vast 'library' of meanings and texts which already exist in culture, and they shape these influences to fuse their own ideas and create a new text. Text producers may be motivated by personal, professional, public, moral, commercial, political, commercial or purely artistic interests and values.

In a public health context, text producers include a vast array of professional health workers, including health practitioners, health promotion specialists, community health workers, advocacy groups and social marketers. These text producers may generate their texts through TV advertising campaigns, pamphlets, petitions, blogs, YouTube videos and animations. Public health professionals also work with professional media text producers in order to integrate health messages into TV soaps, game shows, films and other forms of story-telling.

Non-professional individuals and community groups may also generate health-oriented texts about pleasure and risk. For example, graffiti artists and cartoonists tell stories about the pleasures and dangers associated with certain kinds of drug-use or sexual practices. In many parts of the world, traditional songs and dance have been used by cultural groups to share ideas within their communities about hygiene, family planning and HIV prevention (Dutta 2011).

2. Texts

Texts include every form of mediation that is designed to engage an audience – visual, aural, written. Within these broad categories, media texts may include personal photo images, video, garage music, blockbuster movies, websites, books, Internet downloads, Facebook pages, TV news and so on. Less obviously, perhaps, mediated texts may also include clothing, architecture, dance, art, make-up, jewellery, traffic lights and flower arrangements. Indeed, any system that is structured around communicating something – an idea, feeling or knowledge – can be regarded as a text.

These texts may be broadcast distribution (including global) or narrowcast (including person to person). Increasingly, a vast array of texts is being generated and distributed through the Internet and networked digital technologies, using blogs, wikis, file-sharing and social networking.

Texts are generally created by producers in order to convey some information, idea, emotion or belief. However, as we have noted, there are no guarantees that the meaning that is intended by the text producer will be shared by the audience. There are three related reasons for what is often called 'the intentional fallacy'. First, the actual materials that are used to construct a text – language, tone, images, colour, melody, chords and so on – are actually only symbols (sometimes called signs) which represent the world of lived experiences and things (the world of phenomena): they are never actually the thing of experience itself. This is important point because it means that the language and symbols that are used in media texts are always at a distance from the things to which they refer. That is, there is always a gap between the symbol and the phenomenal world. This gap creates enormous opportunities for variability in meanings and interpretations of any given text. It is part of the reason why 'good health' or 'health risk' might be interpreted in many different ways by many different people (see below).

The second reason for the variability and instability of meanings relates to the ways in which human minds themselves function. While language and symbols are abundant with gaps, so are human minds. Different genetic materials, hormones, past experiences, education, sexual orientation, gender, ethnicity, religion, political background, even where an individual falls within the sibling sequence of a family – all affect the ways in which different personalities are formed and the different ways in which individuals think and interact with their worlds. And clearly, these personal qualities influence the ways in which individual humans interpret media texts and create meanings.

As we have noted above, however, humans rarely, if ever, are able to construct meanings in a social vacuum. Instead, we tend to gravitate towards some form of social bonding and community. To this end, individual practices, values, knowledge and attitudes are generally constructed in relation to significant others and the ways in which the individual imagines himself or herself to 'belong' to a given social group. In this way, individuals generally interpret and reconstruct the meanings of a given media text in terms of their own social reference points. This may be a conscious or sub-conscious process, but in either case the variability in meaning-making is often associated with the individual's sense of who they are, and the values, practices and attitudes that are inscribed through belonging to the social group – whether large, small or a mixture of many.

Not surprisingly, however, the more people who share a given cluster of meanings, the more likely these meaning will be relatively stable and set within a shared knowledge system. As we saw in our examples of Pussy Riot and the British Royal Wedding, mass societies are replete with challenges and reconstruction of meanings. Often, the more people who share a given set of meanings (as in the Royal Wedding), the more stable and durable these meanings become. Even so, these stable meanings may be challenged by alternative meaning sets and marginal groups as in the Pussy Riot political performance art. This move to centrality, domination and control in meaning-making is often associated with powerful institutions (like the British State and Imperial Crown); but challenge and the pursuit of destabilising, new meanings may come from smaller communities, knowledge systems and marginal groups (like Pussy Riot).

Clearly, stability and shared meanings are worthy and productive in some contexts as they enable us to communicate, enjoy one another and work collectively for the public good. In other contexts, however, the stability, durability and power of institutionalised meanings may be unproductive and even harmful, particularly when the assumed knowledge and values restrict debate, challenge and the production of new ideas, texts, values and practices.

This latter scenario is, in fact, a major constraint on social change and particularly social change that supports improvements in health. Old ideas, practices and elite interests may simply lock out new ideas and meanings that will improve a society and its collective of communities. We might consider, for example, the history of exclusion that continued for a long time in the modern democratic state; practices and attitudes that excluded women, LGBTI people, minority ethnic groups and people with disabilities have been dramatically overhauled over the past 30 years through processes of contestation and challenge.

This situation, in fact, refers to the third major reason for textual variability which is directly related to power, politics and the ways in which different social groups seek to impose their ideas, texts and meanings over other social groups. The meaning of texts varies, that is, because they are the subject of what we call 'language wars' (Lewis 2005). This term refers to the ongoing struggles within the mediasphere in which groups with greater access to power, resources and the media seek to override the interests, meanings and practices of others. As these more powerful groups seek to stabilise meanings within knowledge systems that are congruent with their economic, political and cultural interests, the variability of texts and textual meanings becomes tilted in their favour.

Fortunately, these attempts to stabilise and secure meanings so that they become fixed and assumed as social norms are never absolute. For all the reasons we have outlined, meanings can never entirely escape their own intrinsic gaps and instability. Equally, the interests of the powerful groups are subject to counter-meanings that are generated by a diverse array of less powerful, social groups who creatively exploit these gaps in order to express alternative perspectives. As we will explore throughout this book, people are producing, sharing and exchanging texts and ideas about health in a multitude of ways through a vast array of social networks and community organisations. These texts have the potential to challenge orthodoxies and power, explore new possibilities and create new meanings around health.

3. Audiences/users
The 'audience' incorporates any form of text consumer, including anything from audiences of major broadcast media to individuals engaged in online interactions. As we have noted, audiences are far from passive message receivers who obediently reproduce the meanings intended for them by text producers. We couple 'audiences' with 'users' to reinforce the idea that the online and interactive environments facilitate an even more 'active' audience than for a broadcast context – although both interactive and broadcast media engage audiences in active meaning-making. The concept of users simply highlights the rapid role switch between audience and media-maker in an online interactive environment. This role switch also occurs with broadcast media, since most media makers are also audiences at different times. As a shorthand,

therefore, we use the concept of 'audience' to include users of interactive media.

Drawing on the resources of culture and their own personal experiences, relationships and perspectives, audiences actively engage with a text and 'produce' their own distinctive understandings and meanings. Known also as 'markets' and 'publics', audiences create these meanings and re-present them through various social interactions – conversations with friends and family, selection of consumer products, personal style and identity-building, expressions of taste, decisions around their media choices, and participation in social media and online networks.

Many computer enthusiasts rejoice in social media and the Internet as a new text-producing facility where audiences have become increasingly 'active' and are now able to produce their own 'texts', information and knowledge (see Bennett et al. 2011). While certainly the Internet and digital networking systems have contributed to significant developments in media practice, it is simply wrong to claim that audiences were ever passive, or that they were simply incidental to meaning-making processes. Audiences, in fact, have always been critical to the processes and relationships through which meanings are generated. Every communicational act and every meditational text has been produced by a person or group who are also members of an audience. Everything from the clothing ensemble to the blockbuster movie has been made by individuals and groups who are active audiences, people who are processing media texts and their cultural resources to make meanings within the context of their own lives.

4. Culture and the cultural context

While we will discuss the concept of 'culture' in greater detail in the next chapter, it is worth making a few initial comments about the ways in which the text-producer-audience/user interactions are formed in relation to culture. Culture has been defined in many ways. From our perspective, however, it is best to approach culture as the social and political organisation of meanings. Meanings here refers to the ways in which a given social group understands, shares and makes sense of their world.

To break this down further, culture is critical for a given social group's organisation of these meanings. This organisational process is exercised through the group members' relationships with one another and with outsiders. Culture is always political since these relationships are always constituted through various forms of power. Meanings and meaning-making processes, therefore, are shaped in terms of these relationships and their expression in symbols, practice, values, ideology, identity and knowledge systems.

As noted above, however, culture is always in the process of becoming. It is subject to the destabilising and dynamic tensions between greater stability and durability, and the desire for change, deconstruction and the drive to create new meanings.

Culture, therefore, provides the primary resource for the meaning-making that is generated through media. It provides a 'library' of meanings which text-makers draw upon in order to create their own new texts and meaning possibilities. It provides a storehouse of language, images, ideas, sounds and knowledge that the text-producers draw upon. And of course culture is also the storehouse of meanings that an audience/user draws upon to interpret and understand and given media text. In effect, any media text – old or new – is a part of this cultural storehouse. It is an important part of this vast library we call culture.

Cultures, like social groups, can be very large and incorporative, or quite small and highly localised. In modern mass societies, an individual may belong to many groups and hence many cultures, some of which are quite well aligned, some which are quite disjunctive. Consider, for example, the experience of newly arrived migrants who must navigate the dominant culture and its meanings, as well as their home cultures which may be structured around a quite different language, religion, beliefs and practices.

Culture, thus, is an essential part of a given social group's collective memory. It is necessary for individuals and societies to function, share knowledge, cooperate and understand one another. It is also essential for the development of new texts and new knowledge, for social change and the creation of new meanings and relationships.

All of the interactions that drive media and meaning-making, therefore, are subject to the force and significance of culture.

As we can see, the media involves a remarkably complex set of relationships and processes. In the next chapter we will look more directly at the ways in which culture is implicated in these relationships, and in particular the role of culture in the formation and mediation of public health. For the remainder of this chapter we will look more directly at media and public health, using a particular case study to illustrate our arguments.

Media and health

The complexity of the media is particularly pertinent to the broad range of issues associated with public health. As we noted above, 'health' is itself a variable and relative term; different people understand the meaning of health in a range of different ways. While Plato (428–347 BCE) famously commended the nexus of 'healthy mind and healthy body', the Ancient Greek philosopher was really advocating his own version of ascetic warrior exercise and a rather puritanical 'moral wisdom'. Living around the same time, Epicurus (341–270 BCE) challenged this perspective, arguing that good health was necessarily a condition of pleasure of which good wine and good food were essential components.

These sorts of debates and disagreements have continued throughout history and are fundamental to modern lifestyles and various conceptions of health. What is 'healthy' or 'unhealthy' in terms of our minds and bodies is the subject of enormous social discussion, stories, images, information and knowledge. To some extent, these divergent views of what constitutes 'good health' are part of the broad spectrum of individual and group perspectives – the different ways in which people make meaning. As we noted above, social groups construct their knowledge and meanings through their interactions with each other, the media and the cultural ecologies in which they live. For all the reasons we have outlined in our discussion of the cultural model of the media above, individuals and social groups vary enormously in the ways in which they understand health and how they engage with and construct meanings around health.

Thus, the different perspectives and 'language wars' that are generated around health in the media are generally fostered through the interests, practices, values, beliefs and knowledge systems of particular social groups. As we noted, these social groups vary in size, constituency and access to media and other institutional resources. To this end, the meanings that proliferate across the various levels of social life are never evenly distributed; nor indeed do they have an equivalent level of social currency and reach. Thus, the mediation of health issues is never even or consistent across all social groups. Instead, it is subject to interaction with a wide range of competing interests, attitudes, practices and values.

Risk and pleasure

As our reference to Plato and Epicurus indicates, there is a remarkably dense historical and cultural contention over the ways in which health is linked to other critical human dispositions, such as risk, desire, pleasure and displeasure. These contentions very often play at the heart of public discussions about health and the way health issues are represented through the media.

While we might all agree that a bone fracture, lung cancer, obesity and sexually transmissible infections (STIs) may compromise a person's health at a given moment in their lives, the source of this health condition is replete with all sorts of pleasures that contribute to a person's sense of mental and physical well-being in another context or life-stage. That is, the 'risky' behaviour choices and conditions that give rise to injury and ill-health are also associated with a whole range of pleasures and feelings of well-being: a bone fracture while playing sport with friends; lung cancer associated with the pleasures of smoking; obesity from the pleasures of eating rich foods and being physically inactive; or, an STI from the pleasures of unconstrained sex.

Of course, these states of ill-health are both undesirable and preventable. The point, however, is that the various practices and choices that create health risks are often associated with an individual's social and cultural environment and the way that environment modulates risk and pleasure. This is not surprising for an economy that has become increasingly predicated on the production, sale and consumption of culturally inscribed pleasures – most of which are underwritten by, or derive from, the risk of some sort of displeasure. Equally, though, the media is a source of health information and narratives with the potential to facilitate physical and mental health and social cohesion. Thus, while the media might encourage particular kinds of risk-based practices and modes of (over) consumption, it also provides images and information about healthier lifestyles, products, images and practices. That is, the media is not simply a marker of the challenges posed to public health professionals: it is also a facility that enables public health professionals to enter the language wars involved in health promotion.

To put this a little more directly, the media are implicated in:

- promoting particular products, services, lifestyle choices and consumption practices;
- challenging the knowledge systems and dominant social groupings that promote particular perceptions of pleasure and risk that position some practices as legitimate, while others are not;
- presenting information and public debates about health;
  o   priority health problems and risks to health;
  o   causes of health problems;
  o   solutions to health problems and strategies for promoting health.
- mediating between the perspectives of different, and often competing, interests in society (such as governments, industries, health experts and community groups) about responsibility for health problems and strategies for change;
- advocating for systemic political change to address the underlying causes of health problems; and
- enabling communities to voice their experiences and perspectives and take an active role in public decision-making (Dutta 2011; WHO 1986).

Healthcare, health promotion and public health professionals are constantly communicating about health with individuals, communities and society at large. However, this process also takes place against a backdrop of diverse media images and stories about health in popular news reporting, entertainment, advertising, social media and other media forms. These narratives have considerable influence on people's thinking about health: what health issues are important, how other people experience health and illness, what strategies they might use to manage health problems or prevent them in the first place. Through the media, community opinions also influence, and are influenced by, government priorities and policies about the healthcare system and aspects of people's living and working conditions that impact on health. So, it is inevitable that professionals engaged in communicating about health need a sound understanding of the contemporary media.

In the remainder of this chapter, we will illustrate our arguments through a particular theme and case study. First we will focus on the mediation of risk, and then we will apply these ideas to the example of mediated risk and violence for young men. This discussion will illuminate many of the complexities of the media and the ways in which pleasure and displeasure function in the realm of public health communication.

Mediated risk

Risk is an important concept in public health: risk factors, risk behaviour, at-risk populations and risk reduction are all familiar terms for health professionals. A number of social theorists argue that modern societies are defined by a particular approach to risk. Ulrich Beck (2008, 1999, 1992) has argued that modern, global societies have been created through economic, social and ecological risk taking. Societies have grown and developed economically because they have been prepared to take certain kinds of risk. This form of risk-taking by key members of the social group has nevertheless produced certain kinds of 'unintended consequences' – what we have called above 'displeasures'. As well as wealth and economic growth, modern societies have stumbled into wars, internal social tensions, illness, insecurity and severe environmental damage.

Social hierarchies and risk

One of the most important of these negative consequences is the social organisation of citizens through various kinds of hierarchy. That is, modern societies have tended to organise people according to their income, skills, education levels, ethnicity, gender and various other characteristics. While this sort of differentiation has been part of human society for millennia, modern societies have used differentiation as an organising tool that is designed to create greater efficiencies – risk takers in business, for example, will receive higher financial returns for their investment and work outputs; less-risk-taking, low output workers will receive lower financial rewards. As Beck and others point out, this principle is deeply flawed, not only because of the social advantages that undermine fair competition but because the whole notion of 'heirarchy' itself is inscribed with a range of negative consequences. These negative consequences include insecurity, social exclusion, stress, injury, addiction and various physical and mental health problems (Wilkinson & Pickett 2010; Marmot & Wilkinson 2006).

Governments and risk: The information role of the media

Beck and others (e.g. Cottle 2009; Giddens 1990) argue that governments are primarily responsible for managing the 'negative consequences' of these social hierarchies of risk. In democratic societies where governments are elected, this means that the electorate needs valid information about negative consequences in order to elect governments who may prevent or repair the damage. As we noted above, this is a principle function of the 'fourth estate', the news media. According to commentators like Ulrich Beck (2006) and James Curran et al. (2012), governments often fail in their duty because the electorate is deprived of objective and truthful information about their own 'risk society'.

Failing their fourth estate and democratic duties, therefore, the media are ultimately blamed for a multitude of social problems. Simon Cottle (2009) argues that the media promote commercial risk-taking and the legitimacy of differential reward, while also distorting the truth about their negative consequences. According to Ulrich, the media are responsible for the misreporting of social and political issues, leading to a state of 'knowledge, non-knowledge, information and misinformation' (Beck 2006: xiv). Thus, the media are a conduit for both valuable and productive knowledge as well as falsehoods that produce socially damaging effects.

Risk and the mediated 'economy of pleasure'

While Beck, Giddens, Cottle and others conceive of 'risk' as a broad social phenomenon, their theories can be adapted to specific beliefs, values and practices that impact on the health of specific individuals and social groups (Senn 2003; Tulloch & Lupton 2003). As we have noted, modern societies organise individuals into various forms of social grouping. These groupings are based on a range of innate and socially inscribed attributes – education levels, income, cultural practices, ethnicity, physical attractiveness, physical ability-disability, work outputs, religion, locality and so on. Thus, while a 'risk society' may generate various forms of negative consequences, risk practices are also inscribed into the ways in which different groups construct their lives, cultures and practices.

This hierarchical organisation can be either voluntary (people gravitating towards their own identifiable groups) or imposed (modes of social inclusion-exclusion, payment for work, etc.). In any case, the nexus of risk and pleasure is often etched into these heirarchies and their socially ascribed notions of 'reward'. Some very obvious examples of this are associated with different kinds of occupation. Low-skilled occupations, particularly those involving repetitive tasks, heavy labour and lifting, or low levels of autonomy and job insecurity, are also the jobs with highest risk of injury, cardiovascular disease and poor mental health (Brunner & Marmot 2006; Bartley et al. 2006).

Just this simple example demonstrates that the modern 'economy of pleasure' is predicated on a notion of risk which, as Beck and others argue, necessarily implicates negative consequences and 'displeasures'. In a hierarchical system, it is not surprising that those individuals and groups with a higher socio-economic position in society have greater resources available for transferring their 'displeasures' and 'negative consequences' to those people who are more socially 'marginal' or lower on the socio-economic scale. Even so, the individuals and groups who are in these lower ranked and more marginal groups are not excluded from the economy of pleasure nor are they excluded from pleasurable practices and the belief system that propagates the imaginary of risk and reward. Modern societies are replete with pleasures: the whole economic system is based on the fantasies of desire and the possibility of reward for 'risk'.

Indeed, it is important to remember that the differential meanings associated with risk and pleasure are constructed around the ways in which individuals and groups understand and experience their lives. Farmers, construction workers and miners who work in industries with high risk to health are as much concerned about creating positive and pleasurable experiences through their everyday life practices (a beer at the local pub), as the merchant banker, professor or physician (a vintage whisky at the private club). These pleasurable experiences are conjured not by a false imagining or 'false consciousness' (as Karl Marx described it). They are genuinely experienced through the immediacies of their everyday lives and reinforced through various forms of media and media-based stories and imagining.

This means, of course, that there is not a simple, logical or measurable connection between risk and pleasure: rather the two function through various forms of human imaginings. Risk and pleasure are constituted through different forms of recreational practices and the ways in which these practices are inscribed within socially sanctioned beliefs and knowledge systems. While practices like extreme sports, unprotected sex and hallucinogenic drug-consumption may be identified as dangerous by experts and their legal and scientific knowledge systems, these practices are nevertheless inscribed with the risk-pleasure nexus that underpins our economy of pleasure and the ways in which mass society organises and differentiates between people and groups. That is, practices that may appear to be so dangerous to the health of particular individuals and groups are also part of a social system that promotes the social value of risk, even though the rewards of pleasure may be fanciful, distorted or unevenly distributed.

Using the media to influence risk and health: A cultural model

Health promotion media campaigns focus on a range of recreational and work-based risk practices and values. These have included smoking, gambling, excessive consumption of alcohol, drug-use, dangerous driving, unsafe sexual practices, physical inactivity, over-eating and under-eating. Health communication messages frequently point to the negative consequences of risk behaviours, creating messages and graphic images to highlight harmful effects on individual bodies, families and society more generally.

Echoing social critics like Ulrich Beck (2008) and Simon Cottle (2009), health promotion campaigners often claim their campaigns are necessary because these risk behaviours are exalted and glamorised in popular mass media entertainment, news and advertising (Escobar-Chaves & Anderson 2008; Rifkin 2007). Through their powerful story-telling and imagery, the media 'sensationalise' risk behaviours. The power of these images and narratives, that is, entices audiences into suspension of their rational judgement, stimulating a more emotional and sensate engagement with the pleasures of risk-taking.

Escobar-Chaves and Anderson (2008) argue that the media create alluring and often glamorous depictions of risk and danger, engaging the interests of vulnerable audiences, particularly children and adolescents. Smoking in movies, sex and drugs in teen comedies, dangerous driving and guns in action movies are all opportunities for young audiences to vicariously enjoy the thrill of risk. In their review of the psychological literature on the causal relationship between media and risk behaviour in children and adolescents, Escobar and Anderson conclude:

> The largest and most well developed research literature concerns the effects of one type of media content on one type of risky health behaviour – the effect of media violence on aggressive and violent behaviour. That link is

very strong, clearly causal, and surprisingly large. The links between media consumption and smoking and alcohol use also are strong and there is good evidence that they are causal.

(Escobar-Chaves & Anderson 2008: 170)

According to these researchers and many others in public health, there are direct causal links between media portrayals and youth health problems such as suicide, smoking, body dissatisfaction, excessive drug and alcohol consumption and early initiation into sexual activity (Glantz et al. 2010; Goldstein 2008; Pirkis et al. 2006).

These arguments about a direct and powerful causal link between media and young people's risk behaviours can be exemplified in the following cases. The good-looking guy with the sports car and flashy sunglasses can speed through town, beat-up on the bad guys, and win the beautiful woman. This narrative of risk, sex appeal and success, according to researchers like Escobar-Chaves and Anderson, creates an image that other young men seek to mimic. Young men 'identify' with the successful male and seek to imitate his behaviours in order to garner social success. They will drink and drive at excessive speeds, risking horrendous road trauma and death to themselves and others because the media has glamourised these images of youthful masculine potency. Similarly, abundant media images of hyper-thin, fashionable young women create a model of sexual and material prowess that many girls seek to emulate. These media representations of ideal femininity not only contribute to unhealthy body image but also depict a style of womanhood that subordinates women to the fantasies and power of men (Fox-Kales 2011; Wykes & Gunter 2005; Wolf 1991).

Our argument, here, is that the relationship between media and audiences is more complex than this causal behaviourist model acknowledges. Media certainly influence audience practices, attitudes, knowledge formation and experience of the world; however, and as the cultural model of the media demonstrates, these influences work in various directions and through a broad range of relationships and modes of meaning-making. All individuals are constantly referencing to a variety of past experiences, social groups, influences and knowledge systems when 'creating' their own identity, values, attitudes and practices. As we noted in our discussion of the cultural model, humans are not simply passive targets who receive messages or imitate others. The media, equally, is not just a mono-directional system that imposes itself on the thinking and behaviours of individuals and social groups. Media do, however, create opportunities for audiences to reference and refresh their understanding of the world by engaging them through reference to their pre-existing stores of knowledge, meanings and experiences. That is, the representational world of the media is perpetually filtered and re-filtered through the audience member's knowledge bank and the various social groups and contexts to which this audience member belongs.

To this end, the media cannot influence a person's beliefs or practices unless they are congruent with their desires, beliefs and interests and with the conditions of their everyday lives within families, communities and wider cultures. In many respects, this is also the fundamental principle that informs an ecological model of health (Gebbie et al. 2003). Social change cannot be achieved through a simple, causal and linear model of communication or society. Change takes place within a constellation of forces and influences, of which the media is only one. Generating change is not simply a matter of changing or 'reforming' media representations, stories and images so they are more health promoting. Rather, it involves engaging the media in all its varied forms and through a range of different strategies in which culture has a central role.

Mediating risk: Youth and violence

Let's now look at one final example of how the media work in relation to a key public health issue: male youth violence. A number of psychologists, communication and public health scholars argue that the media have a very strong and direct effect on youth and adolescent identity-building and behaviour modelling. The argument is that young people, who are in a transition to full adulthood, are particularly impressionable and hence vulnerable to the images stories and information that are conveyed through the media (DiClements et al. 2009; Escobar-Chaves & Anderson 2008).

According to Russell Viner and his colleagues (2011), the most significant cause of injury and death to young people across the world is associated with transport injuries, violence and suicide. This is especially evident for young men in wealthier, developed countries where the risk of disease, famine and natural disasters has been subdued. According to Viner and his colleagues,

> Violence and suicide became increasingly important causes of death in young men during the study period, together making up a quarter to a third of mortality in all regions by 2000–04. . . . These findings are consistent with country-level reports of rises in youth mortality related to suicide and violence in high-income and middle-income countries during the second half of the 20th century.
>
> (Viner et al. 2011: 1172)

According to a number of scholars, this rise in violent, vehicle-related and suicide deaths correlates directly with the rise of mass media. The proposition here is that modern lifestyles have generated new forms of vulnerability, particularly as young people have become the major consumers of broadcast and interactive media. This 'hyper' connection with the media is rendering younger people increasingly vulnerable to the 'negative consequences' of modern life, including various forms of aggression fuelled by alcohol and other drugs.

This proposition often goes further as scholars argue that the violence of young men, in particular, is directly related to the rise of specific forms of violent media, most recently, violent video games (Massey 2009). A number of quite extensive and well-funded psychological studies have found that playing violent video games stimulates increased aggression in players, creating a greater tolerance of, and interest in, violence (Anderson et al. 2007). Anderson and his colleagues argue that exposure to violent video games 'de-sensitises' players to 'real life' violence, creating a context for mimicry or what is often called 'copycat' aggression and crime.

These conclusions have led other commentators to claim that this desensitisation also conditions citizens into accepting state-sanctioned violence, heavy policing, surveillance and private gun-ownership (Massey 2009). According to Ward (1995), numerous studies also demonstrate that people with high exposure to the prolific violence on popular television are more likely to favour government spending on security, war and the military over measures to prevent violence, such as addressing social exclusion, inequalities and lack of access to education and employment for marginalised groups (see World Health Organization 2010).

Other researchers link violent media, particularly video game-playing, to the psychological disturbances of individual audience members, such as mass murderers like Anders Breivik and the Columbine High School killers (Cullen 2009). Anders Breivik, who killed over 80 people in Norway in 2011, scripted a 1,500-word manifesto on the Internet. In a chilling account of his hatred of Muslims, Breivik describes his preparation for the crime:

> I just bought Modern Warfare 2, the game. It is probably the best military simulator out there and it's one of the hottest games this year... I see MW2 more as a part of my training-simulation than anything else. I've still learned to love it though and especially the multiplayer part is amazing. You can more or less completely simulate actual operations.
>
> (Breivik 2011)

While there have been debates about Breivik's mental health and whether he was 'fit to stand trial', the manifesto outlines a clear and terrible logic to his violence. The video games were not only a source of planning and skill development but also they were a distinct and rationalised 'pleasure', something which Breivik explains as an important part of his mission.

Parenthesising the social and political dimensions of Breivik's crime, media psychologists and public health scholars have blamed the violent video games for the mass murderer's mental condition and excessive violence. Along with the popular media itself, these and other like-minded scholars tend to consider any link between violent media and mass murder as 'proof' of this theory. Thus, the mass murder in Colorado of 24 patrons at the 2012 premiere screening of the Batman movie, *The Dark Knight Rises*, was also considered by scholars and media commentators to add further confirmation to this causal link (R.E.A.L. 2012).

Media violence debates continue to be polarised. For every study that claims to prove causal links between media violence and actual violence or anti-social behaviour, there are others that highlight the limitations of such simplistic associations (see Merrit & Brown 2002). Raul Massey (2009) has repeated a point that has been made many times: if violent media is so dangerous and pervasive, why aren't we all mass killers? The answer to this question relates directly to the points we have been making throughout this chapter. As social agents, we engage with media texts through a range of reference points and the complex web of past experiences, social groupings and systems that contribute to our own personal store of knowledge. We simply don't just 'react' to or absorb the messages the media delivers: rather, we actively construct our own meanings in terms of a broad range of influences, choices and cultural conditions.

Violence is clearly a significant social and public health problem in modern societies. Furthermore, the media are not innocent or blameless in the interplay of social norms around aggressive behaviour and injury (Coleman 2004). However, the media are situated within a complex context of wider influences and engagement. For example, Karen Boyle (2005) argues that the media is certainly implicated in male violence, particularly towards women. But the role of media is more cultural than directly causal: that is, the media is part of a much broader web of knowledge and practices which condone male violence and particular kinds of sexist attitudes towards women. This web of cultural meanings exists within social norms and structures that may include:

- extreme poverty and social inequalities;
- social exclusion and sense of powerlessness;
- the normalisation of violence, in reality, as well as on screen;
- cultures that value assertiveness and aggression, particularly for men;
- the ways masculinity is constructed in a culture at large;
- tolerance of patriarchal cultures and religious codes that sanction the control and discipline of women and children through violence;
- public willingness to consume increasingly explicit portrayals of violence in news and entertainment;
- public support for government legislation that reinforces community perceptions of a violent world, such as liberal gun ownership laws;
- government-sanctioned violence by police against citizens;
- continued support for governments whose policies endorse participation by the military in acts of war and political violence in foreign territories.

Boyle's extensive analysis of the relationship between mediated and actual violence concurs with what we have called the 'cultural ecology of violence' (Lewis 2013; Lewis & Lewis 2012). This is the idea that 'violence' is not a simple action but a broadly dispersed mode of thinking and understanding which informs many of the practices and values that pervade modern societies. This cultural ecology of violence connects aggressive actions and their associated harm, insecurity and displeasure to the broader culture of a pleasure-based economy.

As this chapter has demonstrated, the media is an absolutely crucial player in the cultural ecology of public health, including its knowledge systems, claims, debates and practical actions. But we should not overestimate the extent to which the media is implicated in causing contemporary public health problems; we should also be careful not to overestimate the role media can play in overcoming these problems. By the same token, we should be excited by all that we can do with mediation and how we might work with the diverse array of opportunities that media provide for facilitating health and social change.

CHAPTER SUMMARY

- The media do not simply carry messages from text-makers to passive audiences.
- The media are best understood in terms of the interactive relationship between text producers, texts and audiences.
- Audiences actively engage with media texts through reference to their own experience, significant social groups, knowledge systems, culture, cultural practices and beliefs in order to create meaning.
- It is clear that the psychological approach to media influence and their effects on attitudes and behaviour is limited. The role of media is more cultural than directly causal: that is, the media is part of a much broader web of knowledge and practice that exist within systems of hierarchy and competition.
- These hierarchies and modes of social differentiation affect the ways in which individuals and social groups experience the world and construct their identity, practices, attitudes and knowledge systems through everyday life.
- The media, therefore, do not directly cause risk behaviours and health problems, but they are implicated in these processes of meaning-making.
- Using the example of male youth violence, we can see that the media is just one element within a broader cultural ecology of violence. Simplistic conclusions that exposure to media violence causes violent behaviour overlook the many other aspects of contemporary social life that create the context for acts of violence.
- Health promotion professionals need to understand the complexities of the media in order to work with communities to create communication strategies for health and social change.

References

Anderson, B. 2006, *Imagined Communities: Reflections on the Origin and Spread of Nationalism*, Verso, London.

Anderson, C., Gentile, D. and Buckley, K. 2007, *Violent Video Game Effects on Children and Adolescents: Theory, Research, and Public Policy*, Oxford University Press, New York.

Bartley, M., Ferrie, J. and Montgomery, S. 2006, 'Health and labour market disadvantage: Unemployment, non-employment and job insecurity', in M. Marmot and R. Wilkinson (eds), *Social Determinants of Health*, 2nd Edition, Oxford University Press, London, 78–92.

Beck, U. 1992, *Risk Society: Towards a New Modernity*, Sage, New Delhi.

Beck, U. 1999, *World Risk Society*, Polity, Cambridge.

Beck, U. 2006, *Cosmopolitan Vision*, Polity, Cambridge.

Beck, U. 2008, *World at Risk*, Polity, Cambridge.

Bennett, P., Kendall, A. and McDougall, J. 2011, *After the Media: Culture and Identity in the 21st Century*, Routledge, Oxon.

Boyle, K. 2005, *Media and Violence: Gendering the Debates*, Sage, London.

Breivik, A. 2011, 2083: A European Declaration of Independence. Accessed March 2012   http://publicintelligence.net/anders-behring-breiviks-complete-manifesto-2083-a-european-declaration-of-independence/.

Brunner, E. and Marmot, M. 2006, 'Social organisation, stress and health', in M. Marmot and R. Wilkinson (eds), *Social Determinants of Health*, 2nd Edition, Oxford University Press, London, 6–28.

Cohen, D. 2000, *Yellow Journalism: Scandal, Sensationalism and Gossip in the Media*, Twenty First Century Books, New York.

Coleman, L. 2004, *The Copycat Effect: How the Media and Popular Culture Trigger the Mayhem in Tomorrow's Headlines*, Pocket Books, Beerwah, Australia.

Cottle, S. 2009, *Global Crisis Reporting*, Open University Press, London.

Cullen, D. 2009, *Columbine*, Twelve, New York.

Curran, J. 2011, *Media and Democracy*, Routledge, London.

Curran, J., Fenton, N. and Freedman, D. 2012, *Misunderstanding the Internet*, Routledge, London.

DiClements, R., Santelli, J. and Crosby, R. (eds) 2009, *Adolescent Health: Understanding and Preventing Risk Behaviors*, Jossey Bass, Hoboken, NJ.

Dutta, M. 2011, *Communicating Social Change: Structure, Culture, and Agency*, Routledge, New York.

Escobar-Chaves, S. and Anderson, C. 2008, 'Media and risky behaviors', *Future Child*, 18 (1): 147–180.

Fox-Kales, E. 2011, *Body Shots: Hollywood and the Culture of Eating Disorders*, State University of New York Press, New York.

Frow, J. 2005, *Genre*, Routledge, London.

Gebbie, K., Rosenstock, L. and Hernandez, L. (eds) 2003, *Who Will Keep the Public Healthy? Educating Public Health Professionals for the 21st Century*, IOM Committee on Educating Public Health Professionals for the 21st Century, The National Academies Press, Washington, DC.

Giddens, A. 1990, *Consequences of Modernity*, Polity Press, Cambridge.

Glantz, S., Titus, K., Mitchell, S., Polansky, J. and Kaufmann, R. 2010, 'Smoking in top-Grossing Movies, United States 1991–2009', *Morbidity and Mortality Weekly Report (MMWR), National Center for Chronic Disease Prevention and Health Promotion (CDC)*, 59 (32): 1014–1017.

Goldstein, J. 2008, *War and Gender How Gender Shapes the War System and Vice-a-Versa*, Cambridge University Press, Cambridge.

Lewis, J. 2005, *Language Wars*, Polity, London.

Lewis, J. 2008, *Cultural Studies*, 2nd Edition, Sage, London.

Lewis, J. 2013, *Global Media Apocalypse*, Palgrave, London.

Lewis, J. and Lewis, B. 2012, 'Under the volcano: Media, ecology and the crisis of nature', *Media International Australia*, 145: 50–63.

Marmot, M. and Wilkinson, R. (eds) 2006, *Social Determinants of Health*, 2nd Edition, Oxford University Press, London.

Massey, R. 2009, *The Link Between Video Games and Violence*, GRIN Verlaag, Koln, Germany.

Merritt, R. and Brown, B. 2002, *No Easy Answers: The Truth behind Death at Columbine*, Lantern Books, New York.

Pirkis, J. Burgess, P., Francis C., Blood R. and Jolley D. 2006, 'The relationship between media reporting of suicide and actual suicide in Australia', *Social Science & Medicine*, 62 (11): 2874–2886.

Responsible for Equality and Liberty Organization (R.E.A.L.) 2012, 'Batman movies result in murder – AGAIN – Killing children', 20 July. Accessed 6 May 2014 http://www.realcourage.org/2012/07/batman-movies-inspire-killers.

Rifkin, E. 2007, *The Illusion of Certainty: Health Benefits and Risk*, Springer, New York.

Senn, S. 2003, *Dicing with Death: Chance, Risk and Health*, Cambridge University Press, Cambridge.

The Sydney Morning Herald (SMH) 2007, 'Tragic last words of MySpace suicide girls', *SMH*, 24 April. Accessed 6 May 2014 http://www.smh.com.au/articles/2007/04/23/1177180569460.html.

Tulloch, J. and Lupton, D. 2003, *Risk and Everyday Life*, Sage, London.

Turner, G. 2004, *Understanding Celebrity*, Sage, London.

Viner, R., Coffey, C., Mathers, C., Bloem, P., Costello, A., Santelli, J. and Patton, G. 2011, '50-year mortality trends in children and young people: A study of 50 low-income, middle-income, and high-income countries', *The Lancet*, 377 (9772): 1162–1174.

Ward, I. 1995, 'Agenda-setting and other theories of media effect' *The Politics of the Media*, Macmillan, South Yarra, Australia.

Wilkinson, R. and Pickett, K. 2010, *The Spirit Level: Why Equality Is Better for Everyone*, 2nd Edition, Penguin Books, London.

Wolf, N. 1991, *The Beauty Myth: How Images of Beauty Are Used against Women*, Vintage, London.

World Health Organisation 1986, Ottawa charter for health promotion, in WHO 2009, *Milestones in Health Promotion: Statements from Global Conferences*, WHO/NMH/CHP/09.01, 1–5. Accessed 6 May 2014 http://www.who.int/healthpromotion/Milestones_Health_Promotion_05022010.pdf.

World Health Organization 2010, 'Violence prevention: The evidence', *Series of Briefings on Violence Prevention*, WHO Department of Violence and Injury Prevention and Disability, Geneva. Accessed 6 May 2014 http://www.who.int/violence_injury_prevention/violence/4th_milestones_meeting/evidence_briefings_all.pdf.

Wykes, M. and Gunter, B. 2005, *The Media and Body Image: If Looks Could Kill*, Sage, London.

Culture and Health Communication

3

Chapter overview

This chapter explains the concept of 'culture' and its relevance for health communication. Culture is the clustered meanings that may be expressed in any symbolic system – language, clothing style, artworks, music, architecture, technology, dance styles, political institutions and so on. Put simply, 'culture' represents the accumulated meanings that are available to members of a given social group in order to form their shared understandings of the world. This concept is critical to health communicators as they engage with social groups, their practices and understandings of health.

We illustrate this point by reference to groups' conceptions of health risk and pleasure. While 'culture' is often linked to different nationalities and ethnic groups, it is also highly relevant for almost every other social group. Culture is a crucial concept for understanding the ways in which we interact with each other, the media, and significant fields of knowledge and information. In an increasingly complex, globalising world, social groups and their cultures are understood as being dynamic, overlapping and perpetually changing. This understanding of culture is pivotal if we are to engage with communities in meaningful ways to negotiate change. Culture is the central platform for these negotiations: it is not an impediment, but a space in which we might explore opportunities. Culture is constantly 'in the making' and the media has a central place in the processes by which culture is created and shared, contested and transformed.

Introduction

In the previous chapter we defined the media and the ways in which they work. We argued that media are diverse and complex, and we challenged the idea that media can direct or determine the values, attitudes and practices of individuals and social groups. Meaning-making is generated through the complex relationships and processes that make up the mediasphere. Audiences don't just receive messages and meanings. They interact with media texts and their respective cultures in order to generate meanings, and make sense of their lives and the world around them. In this sense, individuals perform the role of 'audience', 'user' and 'producer' of texts, depending on the given context and media with which they are engaged. While audiences are 'active' meaning-makers, even when watching television or listening to music, they are more obviously active as 'media-makers' when engaging with interactive social media, through blogs, YouTube, Facebook and a diverse array of other social networking platforms.

We also argued that individuals and groups are organised through historically dense hierarchical systems. Our 'sense of the world' is very much predicated on how this world has been shaped through different modes of hierarchy and power relationships. These hierarchies not only work through economic processes and every kind of human relationship, but they are also etched into the knowledge and cultural systems upon which humans depend for their survival, and of course their pleasure and health.

The media and media texts are also marshalled through these hierarchical systems. There is simply no escaping the underlying patterns of differentiation by which given social groups privilege, value and reward particular kinds of knowledge, information or entertainment over others. With their greater access to broadcast media, political and economic resources, élite social groups seek to impose their knowledge systems and meanings over the interests of other social groups. The media, with their capacity to engage and influence a wide range of social groups, are often seen as a key component of these language wars.

Our approach to media and health promotion, the cultural model, expands on older and more linear psychological models of communication. Such models tend to regard the media as the machinery that delivers messages to relatively passive audiences. According to these linear transmission models, audiences are simply the agglomeration of individuals whose personal behaviours and attitudes can be determined and/or changed by media content. Within these models, meaning is relatively unproblematic: audience members generally accept the meanings that are intended by the message senders.

In the cultural model, however, the media text producers and audiences interact with and influence one another and are often in interchangeable roles. The resources that text producers, audiences and users employ for the creation of a text and its meanings are provided by culture. Culture is that invisible but necessary totality of meanings that any given social group regards as its own. Culture is the clustered meanings that may be expressed in any symbolic system – language, clothing style, artworks, music, architecture, technology, dance styles, political institutions and so on. Put simply, 'culture' represents the accumulated meanings that are available to members of a given social group in order to form their shared understanding of the world.

Culture has sometimes been described as 'the web of meaning' which holds a social group together. While this definition might be relevant for older societies, it is less applicable to a complex, globalising world in which social groups and their webs of meaning are very dynamic, overlapping and perpetually changing. Even so, culture is a crucial concept for understanding the world and the ways in which we interact with each other, the media, and significant fields of knowledge and information. An understanding of culture is crucial to our study of individuals and communities, and the ways in which they construct meaning around, and engage with, various health issues.

In this chapter we will look more directly at culture and its relevance to specific social conditions and health outcomes. The chapter will explore strategies that enable health promotion practitioners to work with and through culture in order to engage with communities and individuals around their specific health issues. In the contemporary context, these strategies necessarily involve various forms of media and their meaning-making practices.

What is culture?

We have already argued that culture is best understood as the accumulated meanings and meaning-making processes that are available to members of a given social group in order to shape and understand their everyday lives (Lewis 2008). To emphasise the point, culture in modern, developed societies are far more open and dynamic than older, more homogenous and smaller societies. Humans once lived in relatively fixed community boundaries which tended only to change through the incursion of major catastrophes – invasion, earthquake, drought and so on.

In the contemporary context, with significant flows of people, communication and media across the planet, social groups and their cultures have become exposed to many new influences and forms of mobility. A modern individual, therefore, may belong to many different groups and hence be engaged with many different cultures and potential meanings – social, professional, recreational, ethnic, religious and national. Culture, therefore, should not be considered as a fixed or essential condition, but a relative condition in which the meanings that define a culture are in a state of flux. These meanings are extremely important to any group, but they should not be considered immutable, no matter how ancient their origins.

How does culture work?

The important point here is that 'culture' is neither essentialist and unchangeable nor is it entirely open, arbitrary or constructed. Culture works through a dynamic process that is always associated with a given social group and its claims of 'being'. Thus, culture is always in a state of becoming. It is always dynamic, but this dynamism is always in a state of contention between a movement towards greater stability and a movement to new possibilities and meanings.

As we noted in the previous chapter, meanings themselves are formed through more or less arbitrary relations between words and the things-experiences to which they refer. Meanings, for example, are achieved when social groups establish the use for a word: that use is determined in relation to culture. Without culture, the word has no home, no context for its meanings. When the word or symbol is no longer useful to the group, it either mutates and takes on new meaning and use-value or it simply becomes redundant or disappears. Some words in the current dictionary have clearly mutated from earlier forms – 'between' from 'betwixt', 'afraid' from 'afered' and 'ablutions' from 'ablucions'. Other words, like 'ludibrious' (focus of ridicule), have largely disappeared. Others have changed their meanings or adopted additional meanings – 'gay', 'Black', 'hacker', 'trance', 'mobile', 'social media'. And, of course, a raft of new words has evolved for new needs – 'network', 'Internet', 'transsexual', 'punk', 'tweet', 'selfie'.

As the aggregate of a social group's meanings and meaning-making, culture is, therefore, also the aggregate of change and shifting meanings. Given that social groups are themselves continually subject to hierarchical competition, risk and the pursuit of pleasure, their meanings are perpetually besieged by changing conditions, influences, and internal and external interventions. Thus, while seeking to stabilise themselves and their culture and meanings, social groups nevertheless are subject to a range of destabilising and dynamic conditions.

Cultural conformity

Despite its dynamic character, culture is also the web of meaning that at any given time might be used to support social hierarchies and dominant knowledge systems. As we noted in the previous chapter, different social groups have uneven access to the resources of culture, media and meaning-making. This applies across generations, classes, gender and ethnic groups within a larger society. Unsurprisingly, therefore, in a competition for power and control of social and economic resources, culture becomes a major field of competition. That is, different groups try to impose their meanings and knowledge over others in order to secure the dominant group's social privilege and power. These groups, therefore, seek to marshal culture in order to impose a social order and conformity that is vested in the groups' self-interest and interpretation of the truth.

Even within these standards of conformity, however, individuals may have to navigate different cultural conditions in order to operate in complex modern societies. There may be occasions, for example, where cultural practices of a given ethnic or religious group transgress the norms of more powerful or sizeable groups in a mass society. This is evident where African Muslims have migrated into secular Western states. Particular practices that were acceptable, even required, in the older homeland may well transgress the laws of the adopted state. Such practices range from wearing the Islamic headdress to forms of genital infibulation. While the latter practice is prohibited in Western democratic states, some migrant groups continue to perform female genital infibulation, risking the health of adolescent girls, and legal sanction (WHO 2012; Dopico 2010; Morton 2005).

Culture as opportunity

It is clear that some public health scholars and practitioners tend to see 'culture' as a problem, an inhibition to learning or adopting new health behaviours and practices. While not always explicitly stated, this approach to culture regards certain practices, beliefs and attitudes as 'false knowledge' – knowledge that is in some way deficient or limited by levels of education, ethnic background, class, inherited beliefs, media influences or other forms of misinformation. These sources of misinformation are often linked to 'culture' – that problematic space which has been fixed by history or pre-modern practices and prejudices.

However, rather than see culture as a problem, it is far more productive for health professionals, social scientists and educators to consider culture as a significant resource, the site of possibility, change and renewal. While culture may sometimes defy some of our expert, scientific knowledge, culture also provides pathways to new learning and new ways of knowing the world. Culture, as we have discussed thus far, is a rich and abundant space by which social groups know themselves, each other and the world around them. Its overlaps, instability and capacity for perpetual adaptation and renewal provide new spaces for us to participate in the life of social groups, blending our knowledge and engaging together to generate ideas for improving health outcomes. In the remainder of this chapter we will take some of these principles and apply them to different cultural contexts.

Health and cultural identity

In the context of this discussion, then, we might usefully ask: how are meanings and knowledge shaped around a social group and its shared culture and cultural identity? An individual or group's 'meanings' and knowledge systems may be constructed through a range of human emotions, sensibilities and modes of thinking (cognition). While we often think about 'knowledge' in terms of a body of information that has been logically structured, our argument is that knowledge is just as likely to be formed around human emotions, stories, beliefs, fantasies, intuitions, religion and ideologies.

Thus, while it may seem logical and sensible to invoke expert knowledge systems around health in order to modify health and risk practices of a given individual or group, such knowledge may run counter to the group's pre-existing meanings, cultural knowledge and sense of identity. The issue of changing practices is not a simple matter of exchanging one piece of knowledge for another. An individual or group's knowledge is often embedded in deep history and their sense of identity and purpose in the world – all of which provide a framework for security, comprehension, values and sense of belonging.

The challenge for health communicators is to navigate these various cultural and expert knowledge systems in order to create opportunities for health promotion. This may mean a strategic and sensitive engagement with individuals and communities in order to mobilise beliefs and practices for the purpose of enhanced health. This engagement respects existing cultural knowledge systems and the ways in which communities function.

In one simple example, the authors were involved in a project designed to improve sanitation and water supplies to a very poor village in the northeast of the Indonesian island of Bali. An international Non-Government Organisation (NGO) had provided a new school building for the village. The NGO constructed roof gutters and a large water gathering tank on the side of the school building. It was believed that the capture of clean rain run-off would provide pure drinking water to the villagers, relieving them of the two-hour walk to the nearest community water source. While well-motivated, the international NGO underestimated the Balinese belief system which regards the interruption of water flow as a form of spiritual corruption. Water must be 'flowing' in order to be considered pure enough to drink. The water being held in the tank, which was hygienic and easily accessible, was nevertheless regarded as contaminated and undrinkable. Working with the local community, the authors helped to modify the system so that the water would reticulate in various ways, allowing the free flow of water and restoration of a spiritual purity that was acceptable to the local villagers. While the final result reduced the storage capacity of the tank, the water was now acceptable for drinking.

Social position, hierarchies and power

As we noted in the previous chapter, culture works through a range of social gradients and groupings – from very small and localised constituencies through nations to transnational populations and organisations. We've also established that culture is relatively stable but subject to the ongoing dynamics of change and transformation. Cultural identity is critical to the ways in which individuals and groups engage socially: it is how individuals and groups present themselves to the world.

We also noted that social groups are usually in some form of hierarchical relationship and competition with one another. The history of the world is characterised by severe and often violent competition over economy, territory, resources, knowledge systems and meanings. Inevitably, this form of competitiveness has produced various forms of organisational hierarchy both between individuals in a social grouping and between social groups themselves.

Competition of this kind has contributed to the ways in which societies organise themselves and their meanings. In agricultural civilisations, for example, it was common for the society to be organised very rigidly with marriage between upper and lower ranked individuals being prohibited. Privilege was imbued upon the most powerful members of the society – generally those people who controlled the wealth and military power of a kingdom or empire. In some of these agricultural kingdoms the technology of writing was also restricted, ensuring that only the most privileged people could manage the economic and human resources of the kingdom. Powerful groups controlled

LIBRARY, UNIVERSITY OF CHESTER

knowledge and language in order to maintain their control over economic resources, and vice-à-versa.

This sort of cultural division of differentiation was even exercised through interpersonal communication. It was common, for example, for people on higher levels of the social hierarchy to speak a slightly different language to those on lower ranks. These hierarchical language systems were part of a kingdom and country's laws as lower ranked people were prohibited from speaking the higher version of the language (Anderson 2006).

While many of these forms of legal discrimination have disappeared, most modern societies continue to be organised around the principles of institutionalised hierarchy and competition. That is, societies continue to rank people according to a wide range of differentiations based on income, gender, education, ethnicity, sexual orientation, profession, language skills and even style or 'taste' in cultural products like clothing, music, architectural design and dinner table etiquette.

Social elites, therefore, use culture to fortify their advantage, privilege and power. While this domination is far from absolute, it is nevertheless an important part of the way our society is organised, affecting the ways in which knowledge and information are distributed through a society – including and especially information and opportunities for community decision-making about health.

Dominant ideology and health

This domination-subjugation model of modern societies has prompted many revolutionaries and social reformers to wonder why it is that members of a society are so compliant with their own oppression. To put this in slightly less stark terms, the question might be phrased: how do elite groups maintain their advantage and why is that these hierarchical systems continue to hold their legitimacy, despite the obvious inequities, disadvantages and a competitive system that is far from an 'equal' playing field?

Louis Althusser (2014) argues that culture imposes itself as a false consciousness or 'ideology'. The dominant group manipulates culture so that the group's own interests appear to be the best for everyone. A dominant ideology draws together culturally generated stories about nation, liberal economics, reward for effort and the legitimacy of power. People come to believe in the fantasies that ideology creates, ensuring compliance among the weaker members of a mass society (see Lewis 2008; Taylor 2007; Steger 2002). In a modern Western society these dominant ideologies might include consensus values around 'democracy', individualism, the value of market-based economics, family, monogamy, heterosexuality and even the necessity of hierarchy itself. More subtle aspects of this 'dominant ideology' might include a pride in nation, an acceptance of the need for the military and police, and various rights and freedoms, including the right to access education, healthcare and emergency services.

In health care, the dominant ideology tends to support the primacy of doctors and the system that privileges cure over prevention. Confluent with the belief in the inevitability of hierarchies, this also propagates 'victim-blaming', the idea that health problems are primarily the result of poor lifestyle choices and that people who don't take responsibility for their own health often get what they deserve. Very clearly, risk behaviours like smoking, excessive drinking and consumption of fatty foods are conducive to ill-health. As the dominant ideologies of market economics and individualism tell us, people are entitled to free choice and those who engage in these risk behaviours must take full responsibility for the health consequences. To put it simply, many people in modern Western societies believe so completely in these ideologies, they are never questioned or doubted. They are infused as a dominant and 'normative' way of thinking, even though they may primarily suit the interests of the elite, rather than all social groups.

Public health scholars and practitioners, however, cast doubt on these ideologies, arguing that they often deflect from the real conditions of social life. As noted in the previous chapter, for example, there is clear evidence to show that health is distributed across a social gradient: people on the lower socio-economic ranks of a society have generally worse health outcomes than those people on higher levels (Marmot & Wilkinson 2006). This is, in part, related to comparatively lower levels of education and resources to devote to health and well-being. But as Wilkinson and Pickett (2010) have found, there is now strong evidence to demonstrate the powerful and much more complex effects of social hierarchies on health, including the fact that more equal societies almost always do better in terms of overall health outcomes at a population level.

Some public health scholars and practitioners also argue that people on the higher levels of the social hierarchy actually sustain their privilege through their own vested interests in the propagation of conditions that facilitate these risk behaviours. Manufacturers of cigarette, alcohol, pharmaceutical and fast food companies, for example, reap substantial profits from the risk behaviour of others. Even more insidious, perhaps, is the collusion between these corporations and the mass media. The broadcast mass media generates much of its income through advertising and branding. Advertisers, specifically, rely upon consumer desire to promote sales in their clients' products and services. Media corporations and advertising companies, therefore, are constantly seeking to stimulate desire in order to attract revenue. Profit, rather than good health, motivates the media and advertisers.

In this context, we might consider the advertising and promotion of fast foods that are dense with carbohydrates and fat. While an overload of these foods may lead to serious cardiovascular problems, obesity and diabetes, the foods are usually advertised using various images of attractive people enjoying good health and happiness. Of course, these images don't necessarily falsify the short-term pleasures associated with a shared meal at a fast food outlet, but they do falsify the long-term effects of consuming fatty and sugary foods.

The point, therefore, is that the mass media is implicated in the propagation of particular ideologies and the overall maintenance of social hierarchy. With their greater access to financial resources and capacity to generate and disseminate meanings, the broadcast media dominates our thinking and our perceptions of the world. It enables powerful elites continually to present their interests, stories and political perspectives. In particular, these political perspectives exalt the elite and justify their status and privilege in a competitive and hierarchical social context.

Limits of the ideology thesis

The social compliance-dominant ideology model tends to assume that subordinate individuals and groups are entirely powerless to resist the sources of their oppression. That is, ideology forms a blanket over subordinate groups' thinking and beliefs; there is no escape.

As we have already noted in our discussion of culture, this simply isn't the full story. A dominant ideology and its associated knowledge system is really just the aggregation of a social group's culture and meanings. Like Weber's 'web of meaning' idea, the notion of ideology suggests a complete coverage that allows no space for alternative thinking, challenge and change. In fact, and as we have noted above, culture works in contending directions towards stability and order, and instability and change. The belief system that holds a society together is replete with crisis and contention, fractures that perpetually undermine the stabilising power of social cohesion and stasis.

These fractures in meaning can actually contribute to various forms of social dissatisfaction which may express themselves in various ways. Consider, for example, the Arab uprisings or the London riots of 2011, both of which were driven by social dissatisfaction and a direct challenge to the dominant ideology. Equally, we might consider the problem of mental illness in modern societies. Along with many deeply personal and psychological issues, particular forms of mental illness may also be associated with cultural and ideological fracture. That is, mental illness may have as much to do with cultural dissonance and distress, as any intrinsic or bio-psychological disorder.

If ideology were able to control the thinking of all social actors, then there would probably be considerable uniformity across the various social groups that make up a large society. In fact, there are considerable differences between these groups and the ways in which they relate to one another across the hierarchy. To this end, suicide rates among some groups are higher than for society at large. This is not simply because certain groups are lower on the social scale and deprived of resources for healthy lives but also because members of these groups experience levels of dissatisfaction because they feel less worthy – that is, because the hierarchy and its various mechanisms of social control create as much dissatisfaction as conformity (Wilkinson & Picket 2010). This sense of social alienation and dissonance is often reported in Gay, Lesbian, Bisexual, Transgender, Intersex and Queer (LGBTIQ) communities. Suicide rates are higher for this community than the broader society, particularly during the sensitive phase of 'coming out' (Leach 2006). Suicide rates are also high for groups of long-term unemployed and indigenous communities (Horowitz 2012; Evans 2010).

The point here is that it is the meaning of the social differentiation as much as limited resources that contribute to differences in health outcomes. That is, it is the symbolic status and sense of self generated by being lower on social hierarchies that contributes to particular attitudes, perceptions and health outcomes. In other words, it is how an individual and social group is perceived by others, particularly those higher on social gradients – and how they see themselves in terms of these gradients – which affect a social member's sense of self and self-value.

The ideology, thereby, fractures in the midst of these alternative and challenging modes of thinking. Whether by direct challenge or reactive ill-health, ideology can never entirely subsume or standardise the thinking and experiences of individuals and social groups. Significant as these dominant modes of thinking may be, they are never able to override the instabilities that are intrinsic to culture, language and meaning.

Ideology and cultural change

For many scholars and public health professionals, this social organisation of hierarchy and its continual reinforcement through the media are simply the expression of ideology. As we have noted, the problem with this concept of ideology is the unstable nature of culture, language and knowledge systems which perpetually shift the grounds of social conformity and standardised modes of thinking. Indeed, if ideology worked as a pure state of power, then there could be no space for alternative conceptions, challenge and social change at all. We would all conform and be satisfied with our lot in life.

A majority or dominant culture is comprised of various internal constituent groups and cultures, some of which seek quite consciously to undermine parts or all of the mainstream, and others which merely operate at the margins. Individuals and groups may give the appearance of compliance, or they may comply in certain circumstance; however, they use the spaces of culture to create alternative meanings and practices that are often constituted around a group's own knowledge systems and conceptions of pleasure or risk. There are many examples of this form of explicit or clandestine form of challenge in the realm of politics and social change. But it is also clear that individuals and groups take charge of their health in the context of dominant ideologies. As we will discuss later in the book, there are many examples of health professionals being engaged in health activism and advocacy for policy changes through democratic political participation.

Equally, and in more dangerous circumstances, individuals and groups seek their own health improvement through clandestine activism. Women in Saudi Arabia, for example, have sought to improve their own and their families' economic, mental and physical well-being through a multi-dimensional assault on the country's restrictive driving laws. Legally prohibited from driving, many Saudi women have taken up the challenge of learning to drive, in some cases through disguise and in other cases driving the less heavily scrutinised rural areas of the country. Whether in advanced, secular societies or autocratic kingdoms, the dominant ideology is fractured by the internal dynamics of culture and the active resistance of social members.

Ambiguous culture: Risk and pleasure

While issues of domination and ideology are clearly significant for the health of individuals and social groups, of equal importance are the ways in which citizens respond to these dominant ideas and knowledge systems. Confectionery companies might bombard us with messages and images that encourage unhealthy eating; pharmaceutical companies might exhort us to use their curative products; the medical profession might enjoy a disjunctively high status that ensures we follow this curative model – but in the end, these dominant ideologies cannot compel us to obey. Culture has sufficient slippage, instability and communicational opportunities for us to explore different modes of thinking and alternative knowledge systems.

Culture, as we have already suggested, is really made up of a whole lot of meanings and potential meanings that are not necessarily consistent. As well as its disposition towards stability and conformity, culture bears with it the means of challenge and ambiguity. This ambiguity is especially evident in health issues and the relationship between risk and pleasure.

Thus, the fast food outlets that distribute potentially hazardous fats and sugars are nevertheless an inexpensive resource for the socialising of young people or individuals on low income. That is, the risk of heart disease, obesity and diabetes that might be implicated in these fast foods needs to be weighted against the mental health and emotional benefits that are provided by these cheap food outlets and their products. The same is true of other risk practices, including extreme sports, alcohol consumption and drug-taking (Kuhn, Swartzwelder, &Wilson 2008). While the 'ideology thesis' usefully points to the objectives of elite social groups, it also distracts somewhat from the pleasures that are infused in various risk practices.

Female genital cutting: Cosmetic enhancement

We might illustrate this point by reference to some of the examples we have already cited in this chapter. Consider, for instance, the Muslim migrant groups who continue to practise various forms of genital infibulation. While the participants in this practice may subscribe to many aspects of the dominant culture, they are clearly in breach of the laws that the modern legislature imposes. They are also in breach of the standard norms by which most developed world citizens organise their lives. However, according to the norms of the marginal group, infibulation enhances a woman's beauty, sexual virtue and attractiveness for marriage within the community.

Despite significant legal sanction and attempts to outlaw the practice, these minority communities believe that its continuation is essential for the personal health of women and of the community more broadly. Defenders of the practice also point to the developed world sanction of other forms of female and male genital 'cutting' which are acceptable to the mainstream. Various forms of cosmetic surgery such as labia minora reduction surgery (labiaplasty) and penile circumcision are relatively common in the first world. The incidence of labia surgery is in fact increasing in the Western world, as young women seek to mimic a 'standard' genital aesthetic (Lewis 2011; Braun 2005; Essén & Johnsdotter 2004).

Commentators in Western developed nations who object to this form of surgery usually argue that the 'pleasure' of its aesthetic is part of the media's false imagining, an imagining that has been generated by pornography and its influence on male sexual fantasies (Liao & Creighton 2007). We might also add that this form of cosmetic surgery is part of a more general social and cultural revolution by which casual sex has become normalised and the 'sexual aesthetic' has become more broadly discussed and imagined (Lewis 2011).

In this context, both the genital cutting that is conducted by specific Muslim communities and labia reduction and enhancement surgery are practices that are bound to particular conceptions of beauty, pleasure and social normality. In both cases, however, the female body is central to these respective conceptions and to the ways in which the community and culture conceive of well-being and social health. In both cases, too, the individuals who engage in the practice are referencing to a sense of cultural identity and belonging that in many ways defies the cultural norms and knowledge systems of the wider society, despite their differences in legal status.

In many ways, the female body and female sexuality are critical components to conceptions of a dominant ideology and also to the challenges that may be posed to that domination. On the one hand, it is argued that women are subjected to the dominant ideology of patriarchy; on the other, it can also be argued that women are actually choosing certain kinds of aesthetic enhancement in order to defy the hierarchies that seek to control them. If nothing else, this contradictory perspective and alternative meanings demonstrate the limits of 'ideology' as an analytical concept. While clearly 'ideology' is working through the contending arguments about the female body, these cultural politics are far from simple, settled or one-dimensional. Rather, the arguments and debates surrounding female genital cutting – particularly the comparison between Muslim and non-Muslim cosmetic genital surgery – are indicators of the complexity of culture and cultural politics.

Thus, while it is important to acknowledge that elite and mass groups and cultures can certainly impose themselves and their interests on others and this imposition can have severe negative health implications, it is equally important to remember that the 'ideology thesis' is only one lens, one explanation for negative health outcomes. The very complexity of culture we have outlined in this chapter resists simple or 'binary' explanations of health and the ways in which individuals and groups make sense of their own bodies and the conditions of risk and pleasure.

The role of media representation

To a large extent, risk and pleasure are the core of our economy, our social organisation and our media. Not surprisingly, then, issues around health are inevitably constructed around the same dispositions. We would want to reiterate, however, that risk and pleasure are not opposites. They are overlapping dispositions which are sometimes interdependent like two sides of the same coin: that is, the attainment of pleasure can often involve a level of risk, including the possibility of significant displeasure. Love, the most powerful of our emotional pleasures, for instance, inevitably involves risk of being unrequited, unreturned or being lost. The pleasure of sport involves risk of injury. The pleasure of smoking or eating fatty foods involves the risk of disease.

The ideological model of health often suggests that risk is imposed by powerful groups who prosper from the sale of risky products and services. This binary model places risk at odds with pleasure, often claiming that the pleasures of risk behaviours are largely illusory. It is really only the large corporations and other social elites who prosper from the imposition of these risk products. The media are used to delude audiences into misinformation and false beliefs, leading to an artifice of pleasure in the spectre of danger or delayed displeasure.

From our perspective 'pleasure' is a key component of health and the ways in which the displeasures of ill-health are imagined and conceived. Pleasure is intricately woven into our culture and cultural practices: the difficulty is, of course, that pleasure means different things to different people. Moreover, different people and groups prioritise risk and pleasure in different ways. They place them on a variable scale of rewards. To this end, pleasure is not simply a bodily reaction, the release of endorphins through sensate enjoyment. Rather, and as the French psychoanalyst Jacques Lacan explains, pleasure is an exercise of mind that is connected to these bodily sensations and the stimuli that are generated through culture.

We have already noted that a cultural practice like smoking, which has been directly connected to a range of negative health outcomes, is nevertheless a feature of some form of pleasure. The same may be said of many other risk practices – drug-taking, extreme sports, unprotected sex, consuming sugary and fatty foods. Even practices that deliberately mutilate and mark bodies, such as tattooing, ear-stretching, piercing and infibulation, are often imagined as ultimately pleasurable and 'worth' the pain and risk. From the beginnings of human history into the present, these forms of body-marking and scarring have been seen as emblems of social belonging, identity, status, beauty and courage – the marks of a particular kind of socially inscribed 'pleasure' (Rush 2005). In its most extreme form, even injury and death can be experienced as a form of pleasure. Consider, for example, the satisfaction and 'ecstasy' with which suicide bombers approach their martyrdom. Hideous as we might see these acts, the perpetrators envision and infinite bliss that is reinforced by their significant social group and their knowledge system.

Pleasure, therefore, is clearly linked to the meanings we associate with any given experience. In a complex interaction of sensation, culture and thinking, pleasure and displeasure are formed through a remarkably diverse cast of experiences, practices and knowledge systems (Lewis 2013). Pleasure, therefore, can be defined in terms of immediate bodily sensation as with sexual pleasure, drugs, receiving gifts, winning a tennis match or bet, and various forms of physical activity and exhilaration. Pleasure might also be associated with a more sublime experience, as with religious ecstasy and aesthetics. More broadly, pleasure can be associated with a sense of life satisfaction and well-being. In this case, humans may feel a level of social bliss effected by community connection, identity, life-long romantic connection and family. Very often, these experiences are blended, as individuals engage in various forms of recreational pleasures linked to community and a sense of connectedness. Community drug use and communal dance are very common examples of these cultural practices (Kuhn et al. 2008). Other risk behaviours are often practised in a communal and recreational setting, providing a sense of cultural reinforcement and pleasure to a practice which might seem illogical and dangerous – including infibulation, gang violence, excessive alcohol consumption, drink driving and so on.

The nexus of these pleasures is very often their social and cultural context. As we have argued, it is in the context of culture that the meaning of the practice is assigned and shared. What may seem illogical and even stupid from the perspective of one cultural group and knowledge system, the practice may be entirely normal and pleasurable for another. Health promotion and public health professionals, therefore, must navigate a pathway through these contending knowledge systems in order to work with various communities and facilitate broader choices around health and health outcomes.

Good and bad media representations

In the previous chapter we discussed the ways in which media function. In this chapter we have discussed the role of culture and the ways in which social relationships and hierarchies affect meaning-making. In bringing these two discussions together, we need to remind ourselves that the media are the primary mechanism by which individuals and groups in mass societies talk, know, share information and dispute with one another. The media, in this sense, become a meeting place for members of a social group and society. Taking on their various roles as media users, test-makers and audiences, members of a social group congregate and create meanings and relationships around media and media texts.

Media texts, therefore, play a very critical role in the ways in which we understand and create our conceptions about what is real and true. Texts re-present the world by selecting and arranging particular elements of life-as-lived. These elements are formed into a narrative that accords with a particular media genre – news, fiction, Facebook self-presentation, tweets, musical beats. The audience then draws on his or her own experience to engage with the text and make sense of it. This process of 'making sense' or 'creating meaning' is directly connected to our understandings of truth and reality. The French media theorist Jean Baudrillard argues that we have become so dependent on the proliferating force of media that we are now living in a period of 'hyperreality'.

Things go better with Coke

Whether this description is accurate or not, it is clear that media texts may be regarded as representations of reality. The question then becomes, how well does the text represent life-as-lived? Is the media representation accurate and true? This question is often raised in relation to news and other informational texts that supposedly represent the facts of an issue. It is also sometimes raised in relation to fictional texts and their representation of a given event, person or even class of people. Think, for example, about television and film narratives featuring people of Middle Eastern or Muslim affiliation. Many media critics have seen these representations as false – 'stereotypes' which continually link Muslims to violent attitudes and terrorism.

These questions are linked to the issues of ideology, which we raised earlier in the chapter. There are a number of public health scholars and social critics who remain convinced that the media is insidious and often responsible for engendering health risks and harm through the production of false representations. According to these critics this process of representation can falsify the way things really are, creating a sense of reality that can contribute to negative health outcomes.

In particular, these representations – particularly in advertising – falsify the relationship between pleasure and risk. Advertising continues to confound health issues, as they adhere images of healthy, youthful bodies to products that are known to impair good health. Advertisers never portray Coca-Cola, for example, as a product that causes tooth decay and obesity problems. We drink Coke because it is pleasurable, and because it has been promoted through a social imaginary of good health and having fun.

Pretty woman

More recent examples of public health criticisms of false representation are linked to the female body and 'body image'. Feminists have often argued that the media's obsession with slim, young beautiful women creates considerable disjunction and duress for women who are not part of that minority body-type category (Jeffreys 2009; Wolf 1991). The continual presentation of unrealistically thin female bodies, according to these arguments, creates an impossible ideal for women to imitate, leading to various personal and social crises. At a personal level, this dissatisfaction might contribute to various kinds of physical and mental health problems, including eating disorders like bulimia and anorexia.

On a social level, these types of representation fortify patriarchal ideology and the oppression of women. In her classic study of the 'beauty myth', Naomi Wolf argues that this constant media representation of thin, attractive young women leads to a pursuit of beauty through an obsession with thinness, beauty products and services. The obsession with 'thinness', in particular, has been seen as an adolescence fantasy by which men seek to oppress women by denying their full adulthood. The same accusations have been repeated in the current fashion of female pubic hair removal and genital modification, as we discussed it above.

Very clearly, these images support a multi-billion dollar beauty industry and also contribute to the anxiety and neuroses of many women and men in advanced societies. On the other side of these representations, however, is an historically inscribed social fascination with youth and beauty. Young men and women have been 'aestheticised' across cultures since the first appearance of art in the Upper Palaeolithic around 30,000 years ago. This 'pleasure' of imagining is clearly linked to the human libido and the ways in which desires are stimulated and socially managed. Cultures have always engaged in some form of representation of their significant life events and values – sexuality is a primary example of these representations.

What is rather different about the modern world, however, is the disjunction between the body ideal and frequent representations of both men and women, and significant increases in obesity levels within the developed world. In this context, the ideological argument begins to falter somewhat, or at least expose its limitations. The critique which claims that the media have created conditions of obsessive thinness struggles to explain why this obsession is taking place within a context of increasing fatness and related illnesses – heart disease, diabetes and some cancers. The false representations of thinness seem not to have disturbed the more general reality of our growing body mass in the Western world.

The broader explanation for this disjunction returns us to the problematics of culture and the ways in which modern societies are organised around various kinds of hierarchy and often contending knowledge systems. To put this more simply, we might call these the language wars of the body. Thus, the meaning of the body is subject to the ways in which different social groups pursue their pleasures and seek to mitigate their displeasures within a context of risk.

Groups, sex and culture

To repeat the main point of this chapter, humans seek perpetually to maximise their opportunities for survival and pleasure by referencing to their primary social group(s) and the culture which enables them to make sense of things. Beauty and sexual attractiveness are not universal conditions, but rather they are generated through a cultural group's meaning system. In contemporary societies, fashion and style are part of these beauty factors: a shaved head and skull tattoo may not be attractive to some individuals and groups, but extremely attractive to others.

The same point applies to body size and various modes of pleasure. It also applies to media imagery and the ways in which representations of young female bodies are generated through specific kinds of texts. As we argued throughout this and the previous chapters, the images and meanings that are attached to these bodies are not given or inscribed in the text itself: they are a meeting place in which audiences reference to their group, culture and knowledge systems. While not entirely unpredictable, the meanings that are generated by audiences are fostered around many cultural and personal factors.

In the case of generating pleasure and pleasurable meanings from the representations of attractive young women, audiences may well seek some level of mimicry, but they may equally parcel the text into a broad range of cultural knowledge and practices that have almost nothing to do with trying to be thin or subscribing to a patriarchal adolescence fantasy. They may, in fact, simply connect to other desires, fantasies and pleasures that propitiate sexual activity, self-adornment or the joys of partying, eating, drinking and doing drugs. The media, to this end, is not to blame for any perversion of the imagery or anxiety. The media play into the game of desire within the pleasure economy, but they are not directly responsible for it.

Indeed, even when critiques look in the other direction – towards the media's role in creating the obesity epidemic – the cultural politics of this issue are equally complex. While many public health media campaigns have focused on 'obesity' as a significant health issue, representative members of the community of overweight people have challenged these campaigns, arguing that they are stereotyped and unnecessarily negative. While overweight people have often been the brunt of fictional narrative humour and ridicule, obesity has assumed a significant interest for health promotion aimed at overcoming inactivity and obesity-related diseases.

Trust Jamie Oliver?

These sorts of debates about representation and bodily conditions have been highlighted in recent controversies surrounding celebrity chef, Jamie Oliver. In a series of television programmes and book publications, Oliver has sought to improve the nutritional food choices and food-preparation skills of school children, mostly in working-class families. While generating an interest in good food and a broad-based improvement in school canteen offerings, Oliver has also produced a media entertainment out of criticising the fatty and sugary foods that dominate food choices in many working-class homes and school canteens. Placing families squarely in the media spotlight, he impugns mothers referred to in the press as 'junk mums' who are responsible for children's poor food preferences (see Rich 2011: 16).

As Rich (2011) has shown, some school parents have taken deep offence at Oliver's criticism, arguing that their own social position and privations have been used to entertain television audiences in support of Oliver's own wealth and celebrity status. Others refused to be demeaned by Oliver's on-screen attempts to humiliate them and gathered with placards at school gates handing out pies and chips to their children. In accord with a recent incarnation of political activism around the rights of overweight and obese people (NAAFA 2012), these school parents challenged Oliver and other 'experts' who would impose their knowledge and cultural superiority over a community that has its own values, practices and pleasures.

The point is not that these representations are simply in the 'eye of the beholder', but rather they are set within the complex interactions of culture. Clearly, the school parents have a point. They argue that their life pleasures are being impugned by an external expert system that imposes itself as superior knowledge. Oliver criticises the food choices, without understanding the complex ways in which these foods are connected to the economic constraints, everyday lives, values and pleasures of the people who consume them. Thus, while Oliver's food choices might clearly align with our broader understandings of nutrition and healthy foods, his public health ambitions and media entertainment objectives blunder all over the cultural values of the children and families he claims to be helping. While the programme might make terrific television for audiences who share Oliver's own values and interests, the mothers he has offended clearly invoke a different knowledge system, one that subscribes to different pleasures and practices.

In many respects, this incident illuminates the limitations of a positive-negative framework for health communication. Public health scholars and practitioners often argue that the solution to media narratives and imaging that promote unhealthy behaviours is to discipline the media. That is, the media needs to be populated by accurate information and the 'right' narratives that will promote more positive health behaviours. We might say that this is precisely what Jamie Oliver has attempted to do, though the outcomes were clearly ambiguous.

To this end, the issue of positive and negative representations and the public health professional's engagement with the media needs to be delicately and thoughtfully navigated. It is imperative that we consider the cultural experiences and perspectives of those communities and social groups we are seeking to engage in health promotion. The complexity of culture shouldn't inhibit the possibilities for achieving these objectives nor compromise the integrity of our work. Rather, this complexity should be respected and embraced as having a pivotal role – as indeed should be the people with whom we are working.

Our task as health professionals, thereby, is not to overwhelm the knowledge systems by which others live their lives. Our task is to engage more fully with those knowledge systems, using our toolkit of health communication strategies to negotiate change that may ultimately lead to better health outcomes. Culture is the central platform for these negotiations: it is not an impediment, but a space in which we might explore the opportunities for addressing health problems through a focus on well-being and pleasure. It is the site in which we can work with our communities in order to create new meanings around health through the intrinsic dynamics of human community.

CHAPTER SUMMARY

- Cultural studies offers new ways of understanding culture in the context of health communication by interrogating what culture is and how it is shared.
- Culture is a social group's aggregated meanings.
- Culture is relative and dynamic. It is constructed around stability, as well as a volition towards openness, change and transformation.
- In contemporary societies, culture is constantly 'in the making' and the media has a central place in the processes by which culture is created and shared, contested and transformed.

cont.

- The concept of 'ideology' is often applied in relation to culture and health, although this concept has limitations for a productive understanding of risk and reward.

- It is sometimes difficult to distinguish positive and negative media representations; health professionals need to examine the ways in which these representations function through pleasure, risk and reward in order to work effectively with media to develop strategies for health promotion.

- If health practitioners are to engage with social groups and communities in meaningful ways to negotiate change, an understanding of culture is pivotal. Culture is the central platform for these negotiations: it is not an impediment, but a space in which opportunities can be explored.

References

Althusser, L. 2014, *On the Reproduction of Capitalism: Ideology and Ideological State Apparatuses*, Verso, London.

Anderson, B. 2006, *Language and Power: Exploring Political Cultures in Indonesia*, Equinox Publishing, Sheffield.

Braun, V. 2005, 'In search of (better) sexual pleasure: Female genital "cosmetic" surgery', *Sexualities*, 8 (4): 407–424.

Dopico, M. 2010, *Female Genital Cutting and Sexual Response: Infibulation, Orgasm, and Female Sexual Satisfaction: The Relationship*, Lambert Academic Publishing, Saarbrücken, Germany.

Essén, B. and Johnsdotter, S. 2004, 'Female genital mutilation in the West: Traditional circumcision versus genital cosmetic surgery', *Acta Obstetricia et Gynecologica Scandinavia*, 83 (7): 611–613.

Evans, A. 2010, *Chee Chee: A Study of Aboriginal Suicide*, McGill Queen's University Press, Toronto.

Horowitz, K. 2012, 'Stolen lives? Why aboriginal Australians are killing themselves', *Crikey.Com*, 12 February. Accessed 6 May 2014 http://www.crikey.com.au/2012/02/14/stolen-lives-why-are-indigenous-australians-killing-themselves.

Jeffreys, S. 2009, *The Industrial Vagina: The Political Economy of the Global Sex Trade*, Routledge, London.

Kuhn, C., Swartzwelder, S. and Wilson, W. 2008, *Buzzed: The Straight Facts About the Most Used and Abused Drugs from Alcohol to Ecstasy*, W. W. Norton, New York.

Leach, M. 2006, *Cultural Diversity and Suicide: Ethnic, Religious, Gender and Sexual Orientation Perspectives*, Routledge, London.

Lewis, J. 2008, *Cultural Studies*, 2nd Edition, Sage, London.

Lewis, J. 2011, *Crisis in the Global Mediasphere: Desire, Displeasure and Cultural Transformation*, Palgrave, London.

Lewis, J. 2013, *Global Media Apocalypse*, Palgrave, London.

Liao, L. and Creighton, S. 2007, 'Requests for cosmetic genitoplasty: How should healthcare providers respond?', *British Medical Journal*, 334 (7603): 1090–1092.

Marmot, M. and Wilkinson, R. (eds) 2006, *Social Determinants of Health*, 2nd Edition, Oxford University Press, London.

Morton, C. 2005, *Female Genital Cutting*, Radcliffe Publishing, Oxford.

National Association for the Advancement of Fat Acceptance (NAAFA) 2012, 'We come in all sizes', *NAAFA*. Accessed 6 May 2014 http://www.naafaonline.com/dev2/.

Rich, E. 2011, ' "I see her being obesed!": Public pedagogy, reality media and the obesity crisis', *Health*, 15 (1): 3–21.

Rush, J. 2005, *Spiritual Tattoo: A Cultural History of Tattooing, Piercing, Scarification, Branding, and Implants*, Frog Books, Berkeley.

Steger, M. 2002, *Globalism: The New Market Ideology*, Rowman and Littlefield, Lanham, MD.

Taylor, C. 2007, *A Secular Age*, Harvard University Press, Cambridge, MA.

Wilkinson, R. and Pickett, K. 2010, *The Spirit Level: Why Equality Is Better for Everyone*, 2nd Edition, Penguin Books, London.

Wolf, N. 1991, *The Beauty Myth: How Images of Beauty Are Used against Women*, William Morrow, New York.

World Health Organization (WHO) 2012, 'Female genital mutilation', *World Health Organization Fact Sheet 241*. Accessed 6 May 2014 http://www.who.int/mediacentre/factsheets/fs241/en/index.html.

Working with Media

4

Chapter overview

This chapter presents a guide to modern media and how they function. The chapter is designed to bridge the theoretical discussions of the previous two chapters with the more practical chapters to follow. We begin by outlining some of the ways in which the media can be categorised and used for health communication. These categories include broadcast, narrowcast, community and interactive media. We note that communicators and text producers often use one or a combination of these platforms. Corporate media companies, for example, are introducing various forms of interactivity to their broadcast systems. Moreover, interactive network media systems like the Internet can function as a broadcaster for the delivery of information and texts to diffuse audiences. We also discuss some of the ways in which particular industries, including public relations (PR), advertising and marketing, use these media platforms to provide both challenges and opportunities for communicating about health.

Introduction

In the previous chapters, we have established that the media is best understood as a set of relationships between media producers, texts and audiences/users. We also established that these relationships generate meanings through their interaction with a given social group's culture. Culture is the aggregate of meanings and meaning-making of the social group. Culture and these processes of meaning-making are characterised by opposing forces, moving on the one hand towards greater uniformity and stability, and on the other towards renewal, change and instability.

Our aim now is to demonstrate how these theories work in practice. As we noted at the conclusion of the previous chapter, our approach is to work with the complexity of culture and the mediasphere in order to facilitate communication for health and social change. In this chapter, therefore, we will examine the ways in which various media genres and platforms operate in practice. While working with media will be an important component of the health communication strategies discussed in all subsequent chapters, the current chapter will provide a more general overview of these media and their respective operational opportunities.

Corporate, public and community broadcasting

There are various ways of classifying different media. These classification systems are based on a range of characteristics including ownership, size, corporate style, technology, means of transmission and degree of interactivity. While we will deal with some of the key platform issues later in the chapter, we need to consider first the different objectives and styles that are associated with different kinds of media 'ownership'. These different ownership models have a direct bearing on the ways in which public health professionals engage and work with different media outlets.

To this end, there are three basic models of ownership that apply in most developed world countries – private or commercial media, public or government-owned media and community, non-profit media (sometimes also called 'public' media). We will deal with each of these separately.

1. Private, commercial and corporate media
This category refers to the mass, corporate media, many of which are owned by publicly listed companies that have shareholders, boards and chief executives who actually manage the media activities. While many of these larger media were once family businesses, they have become increasingly corporatised since the 1980s. Rupert Murdoch's transnational News Limited, which produces newspapers, magazines and Internet material, provides services and has subsidiaries in film, TV news, pay TV, rugby, market research and DVD distribution. While constrained in some countries like Australia and the United Kingdom, the Murdoch media empire has enormous audience reach across the planet.

Other commercial mass media companies are less global and may have interests in only one media platform such as newspapers or television. These organisations also have a corporate structure, but they are more narrow in focus and professional expertise. Some of these corporations may have a city or regional focus. Some of these newspapers and other smaller media are owned by families or single owner-operators. These commercial outlets are usually still focused on profit and commercial viability, even though their profit margins may be low and their audience-market share is limited.

Many developing and emerging economies are characterised by a proliferation of smaller news and other media companies. For example, since the fall of the Suharto regime in Indonesia there has been a proliferation of these smaller news and media outlets, as members of the civil society rush to fill the democratic void that was for so long repressed by the authoritarian regime of President Suharto.

2. Public–government media

Government-owned, public broadcasting emerged from the beginning of the 20th century, as democratic nations sought to protect the interests of 'the public' and of the government itself (Miragliotta & Errington 2012; Hajkowski 2011). Recognizing the importance of these democratic values and the need for 'objective' news reporting, governments in Australia, Canada and Great Britain (the United Kingdom) established publicly funded radio broadcast systems in the 1920s and 1930s.

There is considerable debate about the sincerity of these objectives. Some media scholars argue that public broadcasting in democratic states was established to ensure that the interests of the government (rather than the people) were being served. Certainly, the charters of many English-speaking public broadcasters required the broadcaster to support national interests, security, culture and cohesion.

In fact, many (especially conservative) governments in the United Kingdom, Canada and Australia have expressed concerns about the critical nature of their public broadcasters. Journalists, in particular, have often been accused of bias and left-wing sympathies. In this light, public broadcasting news services have been accused of being anti-conservative and critical of liberal, capitalist economics. On the other side, however, progressive liberal thinkers have accused the public broadcasting services of being excessively narrow and limited in vision. Public broadcasting's focus on nation, it is argued, creates a particular bias which subsumes the truly creative, radical, diverse and alternative thinking. Other criticisms claim that the national broadcasters only express a uniform conception of nation, not taking into account the great diversity and multiculturalism of modern nations. In Australia, these concerns led to the establishment of a Special Broadcast Service (SBS) which serves the interests of multiculturalism and social diversity. While beginning as a purely government-funded broadcaster, SBS is now funded through government and commercial advertising.

It should be noted, also, that government broadcasting has a dubious history in authoritarian-totalitarian regimes. Many developing and emerging world countries have strict controls on the media. Along with direct government control, private media are restricted and highly censored, permitting no criticism of government or deviation from standardised national values. China, which is one of the most powerful economies in the world, has extremely strong controls on its media.

3. Community media

In many respects, community media were the first type of media. While community media was initially generated through travelling performers, poets and minstrels, news was often through word of mouth and parish notices. Mass literacy provided opportunities for religious, ethnic and political groups to organise themselves and share entertainments and news through pamphlets and other publications. Today, these forms of newsletters and media are supplemented by broadcast and online systems which have allowed communities to be formed across broad spatial zones and borders.

In what evolved as a kind of non-commercial or 'gift' culture, community media represent a distinct lineage of interests and objectives, many of which are constituted around the cohesion and care of the community and its members. These communities can be formed, therefore, through local, national and transnational communication systems. In the United States the major community broadcast system, PBS (Public Broadcasting Service), represents the major alternative to commercial networked media. In Canada, the United Kingdom and Australia, which have publicly funded media networks, the community media systems are generally local with a very high proportion of ethnic representation. In Australia and Canada community broadcasting is often city- and region-based, though there are also network systems that serve the local broadcasters. Networking systems like the Internet have made it increasingly possible for 'narrowcast' communication and publishing: that is, for members of a given community (including a community of interest) to connect with one another and 'publish' (make public) their information, images and narratives.

The distinctive features of community broadcasting, therefore, include the following:

o   A desire to generate news, entertainment and community-building activities for a given social group. This 'community' may be based on shared values, ethnicity, religion, health experiences, recreational activities, sexuality, political interests, locality and so on.

o   A desire to maintain culture, cultural identity and cultural interests. This is particularly important for migrants and displaced people, but is also true of any marginalised group that feels isolated and is seeking a sense of greater connection.

o   A not-for-profit motive and management system. While some community media are quite broad in reach, others are relatively small. In either case, the primary motive for their media production and sharing is constituted around 'gift' rather than profit.

o   A sense that the mainstream media – both private and public – inadequately represent the interests of a particular community. The mainstream broadcast media may even be hostile to the interests of this particular community and its shared values and interests.

In the past community, media were often restricted by limited funds and access to broadcast technologies and distribution networks. While governments may have provided some opportunities for community broadcast on the radio and television broadcast bands, these opportunities were strictly limited because analogue bandwidth is itself limited and commercial interests generally subsume the interests of community groups. Digital broadcast and interactive systems, however, have provided much expanded opportunities for community broadcasting, particularly through the Internet. The interests of community, therefore, have moved beyond local borders, enabling 'community' to be constructed more easily across the globe.

Broadcast, narrowcast and interactive models

Another way of categorising the various media is through audience size and style of communication. A broadcast mode generally refers to mediation that has a large audience reach. Perhaps the most spectacular example of this broadcast model at work was the Royal Wedding in 2011. An estimated three billion people across the planet watched the wedding of Prince William and Kate Middleton (Lewis 2013). Very clearly, this vast number of viewers included people from very different backgrounds and with remarkably different values and lifestyles. The uniting characteristic, we might assume, was an interest in love, pageant, celebrity, glamour and youthful beauty.

While such a large audience is unique, mass broadcasting generally seeks to attract an audience which will generate and maximise profit. This profit may be generated through the direct purchase of a media product – ticket sales at a concert or movie, newspapers, DVDs or other merchandise. It may also be through advertisers paying to access a given audience, as is often the case with commercial TV. In this case TV stations purchase a programme from its producers and then on-sell access to advertisers who want to promote their products on behalf of clients. Generally, the more popular a programme is with an advertiser's target market, the higher the price they will pay.

In general, advertisers seek access to that group of a society's income earners who are most likely to purchase their client's products or services. Often advertisers use a five-part scale to describe and define a given national society: Group A is those people who are the smallest proportion of the wealthiest people in a society; at the other end of the scale, Group E is the poorest of unemployed and marginal people; the middle groups are usually referred to as 'aspirational', people who are employed and who are seeking to improve their material lives through income earning and spending. It is these groups that the advertisers are usually seeking to target on behalf of their clients.

Advertisers and PR companies will also pay for access to smaller audiences, provided they are of particular interest to the clients and their products and services. The concept of narrowcasting has been applied to these smaller, more homogenous audience groups. The idea here is that the media producers focus their text on the particular nuanced interests of a given social group. On Pay TV, for example, there may be a specific recreational activity that attracts a small but highly focused audience group – dirt bike riders, for example. Advertisers of products that will interest this group will pay for access on behalf of the manufacturers of these bikes, activities and related products.

Even within the broadcast system, therefore, we may have media texts that are highly targeted. Hence we will have 'art-house' films or films that will have limited distribution through special interest outlets. Surf movies, for example, were originally distributed through town halls in coastal areas; they are now sold as DVDs in surf retail stores and distributed online. Similarly, many other community texts are distributed through community radio or TV broadcast systems.

Perhaps the narrowest form of all media is through various forms of interactive communication systems. Evolving through telegraphy, telephony and data storage frames, the Internet is the most flexible of these narrowcast and interactive systems. While we will say a little more about this in subsequent sections, it is important to note that the Internet and computer-mediated communication systems are hybrid media forms which can be 'broadcast', 'narrowcast' and 'one-to-one' communication. As a convergent facility that draws together a very broad range of mediation technologies and services, the Internet enables communication between people on the next desk, across the city, nation and the globe.

This flexibility enables users to generate their own texts, some of which can become 'viral' and reach millions of audience members through Web 2.0 technologies via YouTube, blogs and diverse array of social media platforms. Equally, however, social networking systems like Facebook and MySpace can be used to generate texts that are shared among niche audiences that are very small but interested in specific issues and content.

At the same time, major media broadcasters have also invaded the Internet, using its network systems to enhance their existing texts and create feedback loops with audiences and readers (Castells 2009). While seeking to find a sustainable financial model, most of the world's major newspapers have established an online presence. In the midst of a rapid expansion of blogging, community-generated news and citizen journalism, the commercial media are seeking strategies to reassert their professional and social authority among this flush of various narrowcast and interactive news systems.

Convergence and digital networked media

The name that is usually given to this changing media environment is 'convergence'. Most often, this term refers to the convergence of previously distinctive media platforms – TV, radio, print, telephony – into an integrated multi-platform system. While there is no doubt that traditional media platforms continue to have significant audiences and social appeal (television, radio, print), the Internet and other digital systems are creating a new technological apparatus and system for different kinds of media experience. Again, as we understand the media to be a set of relationships, the Internet enables these relationships to construct new pathways and practices for textual production, sharing, audience engagement and meaning-making.

While we will talk about the many recent developments in using interactive media for health communication in the course of later chapters, it is important to note here that there is considerable enthusiasm for the interactive media among many public health professionals, as it provides facilities for navigating pathways for direct engagement with target audiences. In particular, many health promotion practitioners see the Internet as a space through which they can evade the costs and controls of broadcast systems and communicate more directly with target communities and audiences. Moreover, the Internet enables individuals and communities themselves to talk to one another, share information and even access professional knowledge without the intermediary of high-cost and sometimes confusing medical experts and their vested interests.

This community narrowcasting and interactivity is a feature of what has been called Web 2.0 or the 'social web'. Emerging in the early 2000s, this form of social networking has been generated by the altruistic and community gift culture that inspired many early Internet utopians (e.g. Turkle 1997; Rheingold 1993). The notion of a social media as Web 2.0 emerged after the infamous tech-bubble crash of the late 1990s. The second-coming of the Internet, according to the enthusiasts, was generated through this new form of knowledge sharing and community-building (Lewis 2008; Solomon & Schrum 2007). Facebook, YouTube, Twitter and innumerable other interactive systems supported these ideals, creating a space for the free sharing of information and creative texts.

Thus, older information and broadcast systems deploy expensive production and transmission technologies, disposing them to high investment and profit business models. Computer-mediated communication systems, on the other hand, have evolved relatively inexpensive technological systems which enable low-cost production and dissemination of texts. The Internet and World Wide Web, thereby, enable users to by-pass corporate information systems, enabling direct access and participation in the global mediasphere. As we will explore throughout later chapters, Blog-worlds, Second Life, wikis and the broad range of social media platforms have vastly expanded opportunities for users to connect with one another through networked systems.

These opportunities are particularly important for public health professionals who are seeking to communicate with communities and individuals beyond the borders of corporate media. Digital and social media allow public health professionals to narrowcast health information and reach audiences more effectively. Internet and social media also create valuable opportunities for collaborating with individuals and communities to identify needs, develop communication strategies and disseminate them within their communities. This is particularly important when working with marginalised groups such as minority ethnic or religious groups and people with disabilities, chronic illness or stigmatised conditions, and more marginal or sensitive issues, such as IV drug use, genital infibulation, domestic violence, and explicit sexual health information for sex workers and LGBTI communities (Pullen & Cooper 2010).

Moreover, and as we discussed in the previous chapters, the mass media are often tied to other commercial products and services, which may have negative implications for people's health. Public health professionals have an important role in countering the marketing of potentially harmful products like tobacco, alcohol, low-nutrient processed foods and unsafe consumer products, by raising awareness about the risks to health and how these may be minimised. As we will see in Chapter 6, the Internet, social media and other Web 2.0 technologies have proven to be extremely effective tools in public health 'counter-marketing' to subvert the powerful influence of commercial marketing and advertising industries. In the United States, the United Kingdom and Australia for example, counter-marketing has undermined the reputation of the world's biggest tobacco companies, exposing unethical marketing strategies and challenging the corporate vested interests who benefit from the sale of tobacco products that cause death and chronic disability for millions of people every year worldwide.

Advertising and public relations

As we discussed in chapters 2 and 3, pleasure is a critical component of human life: advertising, marketing and PR firms know this better than anybody. As we have noted, advertising is a key part of the business model of commercial media. This connection between media and advertising is quite explicit in the newspaper, radio, television and Internet media industries where advertising revenue is a major part of a company's income stream. In movies and even the popular music industry, however, advertising is also very important, particularly through strategies like product endorsement, merchandising and product placement. In the James Bond movie, *Quantum of Solace* (2008), for example, the film producers invited automobile manufacturers to bid for their car to become the new James Bond super-auto. Seeking to re-tag the Volvo's image as a reliable and safe family car, the Volvo company outbid its rivals as they sought to attract a younger and more racy market.

Both media information and entertainment industries are clearly bound to this sort of social imaging and consumer pleasure. Indeed, while pleasure has always been a part of human social organisation and culture, the emergence of consumer society through the late 19th and early 20th centuries marked a major amplification of an economy of pleasure. The development of mass media was a critical component of this new consumerism. Advertising, marketing, branding and PR evolved as the commercial conduit that connected the creative and information industries with the broader consumer economy.

To put it simply, consumer society is marked by a significant shift in the way capitalist economics work. While earlier societies, including earlier capitalist societies, were organised around the production and sale of things that people need, consumer capitalism has been constructed around the things that people 'desire' – that is the things that bring pleasure over necessity (see also Lewis 2010; Humphery 2010; Baudrillard 1998). Thus, while people might need food, clothing and shelter, only the wealthy people in the past could afford decorative clothing, luxurious houses, holidays and exotic foods. Having satisfied these basic needs, capitalist economies continued to grow through the expansion of demands and desires. Through the combination of greater social wealth and the techniques of mass production, more and more products became available to greater numbers of people. This growth trajectory has been built around the ceaseless expansion of consumer desire and conceptions of pleasure.

While many media businesses were constructed around the production of news, information and narrative fiction, advertising and PR were directly engaged in the commercial production of desire. Adapting the methods of narrative story-telling and the arts, advertisers enhanced the purpose ('use-value') of a given product through an attachment of symbols, design features, images and narratives. That is, they enhanced the consumer interest in and desire for a product or service through the addition of 'symbolic value'. This symbolic value added meaning that radically supplemented the use-value of the product. Marlboro cigarettes were enhanced by the narrative of a rugged, good-looking horseback cowboy; automobiles were enhanced by the admiration of a beautiful young woman; McDonald's hamburgers were drenched in colour, a happy clown and thriving family.

Using the mass media to promote their clients' products, the advertisers created a narrative fantasy that would stimulate the consumer's interest and desire to buy. Product manufacturers and service providers use advertising companies to optimise their market advantage and hence their profits. Very often, too, manufacturers and service providers will employ marketing companies and PR companies to create a more generalised aura and image around their products and services. This image or public perception of the product is generated around what is called 'brand'. This brand is something more than just a specific advertising campaign but is more complete, an accretion of longer term promotion, advertising and corporate image-building strategies. These strategies include sponsorship of artistic and sporting events, charity and other forms of civic participation.

Within a highly competitive marketplace, this branding enables the product to be identified in the imagination and thinking of the consumer. As we noted, if the product or service has some form of health risk attached to it, then the PR and marketing companies have to work even harder to ensure a positive public conception of the product: they must realign people's thinking somehow in order to parenthesise or re-inscribe the public's perception of this risk.

In his book, *Toxic Waste Is Good for You*, John Stauber (2002) argues that PR companies work very hard to create the image of corporate social responsibility through the manipulation of news and other media information systems. Thus, while most people recognise advertising as a clear enhancement of a product's qualities, there appears to be far less public awareness of the ways in which PR professionals manipulate product branding and public perceptions through more surreptitious means.

Through various strategies, PR professionals infiltrate the mediasphere, seeking to create a positive public image for clients and their products. PR and marketing are not of themselves unethical or inimical; indeed, the same strategies can be used to promote products and services that may generate negative as well as positive health outcomes. In a context of economic competitiveness and cultural contest, public health professionals must deploy equally compelling strategies in order to expose the risks and challenge the health information generated through PR and marketing companies.

While these strategies and many others will be discussed in the following chapters, it is important to remember that 'the media' is a central battlefield in these PR wars. We can summarise some of the strategies that PR and marketing companies deploy in the promotion of their clients' interests as follows:

1.   direct advertising campaigns;
2.   sponsorship of significant cultural events in sport and the arts;

3. sponsorship of education and civic programmes, including scholarships and exchange programmes;
4. charity and support of good causes;
5. engaging celebrities as spokesmen and women;
6. generating artificial activity and interest in a client or client's product through social media ('astroturfing');
7. constructing an impression of social interest and activity through media seeding on talk-back radio; individuals are paid by the PR company to act like random callers;
8. preparation of 'media-releases', news stories and film footage which are submitted to news organisations and TV studios for public release;
9. lobbying government and politicians through various strategies, including email bombing, petition, high level meetings, and electoral publicity.

As noted, many of these strategies will be discussed during the course of the next chapters.

Public relations, governments and public health

Public health professionals need to be aware of some of the less visible strategies that are employed by PR processes in the areas of health. Government lobbying is one of the more contentious processes by which PR and marketing companies seek to influence public policy and hence various health outcomes.

In order to enhance and protect a product or service brand, PR companies often seek to influence government policy and regulatory processes. As we know, democratic governments have only delegated power and are 'responsible' to the interests of their citizens. This principle of 'responsible government' generally implies the provision a range of services to ensure the well-being and security of the people. These services include military and civil security, education, infrastructure, economic management and of course health. Clearly, we expect our governments to protect us and ensure that other society members do not inflict harm on us.

This role extends to the protection of citizens from potentially harmful products and services. This responsibility, however, at times may run counter to other governmental responsibilities, including provision of security and economic management. For example, recruiting soldiers and sending them to war is clearly a risk activity, but governments sacrifice the health of some citizens in order to protect the well-being, health and security of others.

Equally, in a liberal capitalist system individuals and organisations require a certain level of freedom to produce products and services that are devoted to pleasure. Where these pleasures may also elicit displeasure and health damage, governments must determine the level of 'acceptable' risk and how to manage vulnerability. To this end, governments may need to intervene in the commercial process, even where there is clear demand for these potentially harmful products and services.

The principal techniques for managing this balance include the following:

1. Prohibition: the complete ban on substances at production, sale and consumption. This is the tool that is used, for example, with some forms of recreational drugs and child pornography. It is also the tool used for products that are retrospectively found to be harmful such as asbestos and pharmaceuticals like thalidomide.
2. Regulatory controls on sale, advertising, distribution and consumption of potentially harmful products. Tobacco is the most obvious of this form of regulation where sale is restricted to younger people and there are controls on where smoking can occur.
3. Health promotion campaigns. Where governments have identified health problem such as smoking, AIDS or obesity, they have sponsored public education and awareness campaigns in order to shift citizens' attitudes and behaviour.
4. Taxes and fiscal management of companies that produce harmful products. Again tobacco and some forms of alcohol are heavily taxed in order to deter sales. These tax revenues are sometimes re-directed towards health promotion.

Of course, governments have many priorities and are involved in complex modes of political, economic and social judgement. Not surprisingly, therefore, health advocates are often engaged in lobbying governments in order to shift these priorities in favour of the public interest. Once again, these forms of lobbying may be exercised on behalf of clients who produce potentially harmful products and services, or on behalf of communities and public interest organisations who are seeking better health outcomes.

Corporations, in particular, often form industry-based lobby organisations or hire PR firms to present their cases to governments and the citizens. PR companies, as noted above, use the mass media to support their claims, often generating news releases and well-packaged materials for direct supply to news organisations. James Curran (2011; Curran et al. 2012) argues that news organisations have, in fact, come to rely on these PR news feeds over the past several decades, largely because they have lost much of their professionalism and financial integrity. According to Curran and many other media scholars, this financial vulnerability occurred through the impact of commercialisation and globalisation during the 1980s. Following the high point of media professionalism, Curran claims, media organisations became subjected to intense corporate speculation, and buying and selling on the stock market. The media became more corporatised and exposed to these corporate raiders who stripped away their professionalism in order to reduce costs and produce cheaper global media product.

Clearly, one of the cheapest ways to produce print or TV news is to gather stories from free sources. In this cultural and economic environment PR companies could generate stories around products and services and provide them free-of-charge to the news organisations. The news organisations would then present the material as objective and true for distribution to their audiences. News and media stories that have these sorts of bias inscribed in them have considerable potential to influence some of the public's meaning-making and view of various social issues. Governments, which are sensitive to public opinion, are therefore more likely to respond by adjusting public policy.

This sense of social and public interest in a given topic is also being generated through the Internet and especially social media. As democratic governments seek to respond responsibly to public interests and priorities (and therefore stay in power), they are increasingly reacting to 'activity' in the Internet environment, as well as to the mass media. Increasingly, PR and marketing companies are using social media to generate a sense of public interest and activity. In particular, the strategy of 'astroturfing' has been adapted to the Internet, as PR companies have recognised the ways in which publics, mass news organisations and governments use social media as an indicator of public opinion (Monbiot 2011). The concept of astroturfing derives from the idea that astroturf is an artificial grass surface: PR companies have evolved various practices and mechanisms for giving the impression that a particular policy, product or idea attracts strong public support.

Using older broadcast media and various forms of PR strategies during the 1980s, tobacco companies were particularly active in generating an impression of public support (Tobacco Tactics 2011; Freeman & Chapman 2010). While they are now prohibited from broadcast advertising in much of the Western world, many tobacco companies are using YouTube, Facebook and other social media to generate online activity that gives an impression of public interest and approval of their products. This model is now stock-in-trade for a range of corporations, propagandists, political lobbyists and public authorities. Indeed, a whole new generation of activists, professional media workers and software applications have evolved around social media and the 'impression' of public activity. In particular, these individuals and groups generate a range of texts that are published in the blogosphere, social networking sites, YouTube and a range of online forums. While these social media sites are often designed around the everyday social media users, activists and professionals invade the sites with very specific political or commercial purposes.

One of these strategies is to generate false identities of 'persona', releasing that imagined person (astroturfers) into various forms of social media activity. George Monbiot (2011) describes the use of specifically designed 'persona management' software which multiplies the identity of astroturfers on a site, creating the impression of popular activity around a significant issue. Listing their interests through Facebook and other sites, the astroturfers are able to populate a given political zone: 'Fake accounts can be kept updated by automatically reposting or linking to content generated elsewhere, reinforcing the impression that the account holders are real and active' (Monbiot 2011).

Governments and the military are also engaging in this practice as they seek to engender public support and interest in particular policies and activities. According to Monbiot, the US military, in particular, is recruiting software companies to support various astroturfing activities, particularly around restrictions on civil freedoms and the necessity for public surveillance in a time of increasing global insecurity.

Industries and influence: Pharmaceutical and other health stories

Many public health policy interventions involve changing laws, regulations, policies, taxes, prices and product standards. These public health initiatives are often opposed by various elements of government, industry and even other health sectors concerned about changes to policies and regulations that could potentially work against their interests. Within this context, public health advocates must compete for prominence in a highly contested political arena – often in the face of well-resourced and highly organised opposition. This means that advocates for public health initiatives also need to make strategic use of the media to influence news coverage, public discussion and political debate in order to influence the decision makers with responsibility for laws, regulations or policies that affect health.

This is not only critical for challenging the information that is being marshalled by the producers of potentially harmful foods, beverages, other substances and services, but it is also important for engaging with the providers of medical services and health-related products that carry potential risks and harm. In a society and economy that is largely predicated on the commercial transaction of pleasures, it is not surprising that many products have been created around the prevention of displeasure. Inevitably, the perpetual stimulation of desire for pleasure is predicated on some level of dissatisfaction and the avoidance of displeasure. Providers of particular products and services seek, therefore, to stimulate displeasure in order to sell a solution or cure. Naomi Wolf (1991) has argued that this stimulation of displeasure is a key driver of the cosmetics industry. It is also clearly implicated in various forms of eating disorder where young people, in particular, feel a high level of dissatisfaction with their appearance and body image (Maine & Kelly 2005).

As it is described in the film *Love and Other Drugs* (Edward Zwick 2010), this level of dissatisfaction is also a key driver of the pharmaceutical industry. While clearly there are many prescription drugs that have benefited many people, there are also many drugs that are either harmful or unnecessary. Pharmaceutical companies have become major players in the PR industry, identifying health conditions that only their newest and greatest drug may cure.

Critical commentators such as Moynihan and Cassells (2005) have provided illuminating research to expose the strategies used by some of the world's biggest drug companies to systematically contribute to the medicalisation of ordinary conditions, widen the boundaries that define illness and increase the markets for medication. Mild problems become redefined as serious illness and common complaints are labelled as medical conditions requiring drug treatments. By widening the boundaries of illness and lowering the threshold for treatments, the pharmaceutical industry is creating millions of new patients and billions in new profits, in turn threatening to bankrupt healthcare systems in many countries.

Numerous industries benefit from expanded markets for tests and treatments (including drugs) and pharmaceutical industries have wide-reaching influence within the medical and healthcare professions. Driven by their vested interest in overdiagnosis, these companies provide funding for direct-to-consumer advertising; establish research foundations to provide evidence supporting their products; sponsor medical education; and conduct strategically targeted 'disease awareness' campaigns through news and current affairs. These industries also exert their influence by sponsoring a wide range of online forums, support groups and patient communities, often using astroturfing to feed into online discussions in ways that promote their corporate interests. Not surprisingly, many of these sponsored groups tend to be quick to celebrate new treatments and technologies but much slower to publicly criticise their limited effectiveness, excessive cost or less publicised side effects (Moynihan & Mintzes 2010).

Moynihan and colleagues (2012) demonstrate how this cycle of overdiagnosis feeds into deep cultural norms that more 'medicine is better'. The authors cite recent evidence to suggest that patients tend to report greater satisfaction when they have increased access to tests and treatments, even though more care may be associated with greater harm. Evidence is mounting that overdiagnosis and associated risks pose not only a serious threat to human health but also undermine the rational use of public resources. For example, the cost of unnecessary treatments in the United States is over US$200 billion which could be more effectively used to help those people in serious need of medical care.

Interactive media and public health communication

We have discussed the interactive networked media throughout this chapter, largely as a component of all media activities and industries. All media industries use a combination of media platforms to distribute their texts. These media platforms may be broadcast, narrowcast or interactive in their general orientation. Broadcast media corporations are using various forms of interactivity to connect more strongly with their markets/audiences. Similarly, community organisations and narrowcasters often use the Internet for both interactive and certain kinds of narrowcasting. The Internet can also be used in certain circumstances as a broadcast system – it allows us to deliver texts and information to wide audiences. There are many YouTube videos, for example, that have had well over 100 million views.

Thus, it is no longer possible to draw clear lines between 'old' and 'new' media, or even digital and analogue media, since so much mediation is now digitally composed and distributed. Even so, it is critical for health communicators to engage with the interactive networked media which is an extraordinarily accessible medium in the developed and emerging worlds.

Networked digital technologies and the convergence of the media industries are radically shifting the ways in which the media function. This dynamic and interactive media environment is altering media production, distribution and consumption. There are now many forms of media other than corporate mass media that influence people's attitudes and values about health. In some instances, audience groups are becoming smaller and more concentrated as they select media content to suit their tastes and preferences. Web 2.0 technologies are enabling people to collaborate and share information as they interact, create new content and share it with others of similar interests and social connections. A vast array of communities are creating their own ways of communicating about themselves and their issues, creating stories, sharing them and opening up their perspectives to the wider global community.

Within this context, health communication is no longer assumed to be a top-down, expert-led process of developing targeted messages to change the beliefs and practices of individuals. Instead, people and communities are becoming agents of change through their engagement with – and influence on – various media and emerging modes of communication. The Internet and interactive digital media are creating a plethora of opportunities for social networking and community-building, development, community mobilizing, advocacy and activism for health and social change (Dutta 2011; Pullen & Cooper 2010).

According to Lefebvre (2013), interactive media create a wide range of opportunities for health communication to move away from its traditional focus on 'messages and target audiences' to become more involved in the following:

- Enhancing existing linkages between people and communities, not only to share knowledge and resources but also to deepen and strengthen support between people trying to create positive social change.
- Nurturing and sustaining new types of linkages that bring people together around similar interests, a shared 'mission' or addressing a common problem.
- Better engaging communities in problem-solving by creating new networks of people supporting community-level change.
- Weaving together existing networks of groups not normally accustomed to working together to create new sources of inspiration and power to address health and social issues.
- Engage communities in new ways to mobilise and to engage with priority public health issues.

These issues will be taken up and discussed in greater detail each of the practical chapters throughout this book.

Interactivity: Some debates and doubts

Interactive media presents enormous opportunities and advantages for health communicators. However, there are also some important issues and consequences associated with the interactive media that are not always acknowledged by network and social media enthusiasts. While we will explore these issues in subsequent chapters, they can be summarised as follows:

1. Social media has become increasingly invaded by PR and other lobby groups who are not always honest about the identities they are creating nor about the products, people and events they are promoting (Stoff 2008).
2. While information is readily available through the networked system, much of this information is untrustworthy or just plain inaccurate (McChesney 2013).
3. The most viewed and read sites on the Internet are generated by broadcast and corporate organisations. As well as Google, YouTube and Facebook, the sites that are most often read for information and entertainment are also owned by large media organisations like the Huffington Post, CNN and the New York Times (Ebiz 2013).
4. Even the most read bloggers on the Internet are typically professional journalists and academics, rather than the amateur enthusiast (Ebiz 2013). Thus, the idea that the Internet is a fundamentally equal or democratic space is not supported by this imbalance. As Matthew Hindman (2009) argues, there is a huge difference between being published on the Net, and actually being read.
5. Increasingly, it is also being claimed that social media provides a platform for the expression of loneliness more than friendship. Sherry Turkle (2011) describes this experience as being 'alone together'. Her research explores the social implications of technology-dependent relationships at the expense of real-life human expressions of caring, intimacy and trust.
6. The rise of citizen journalism and crowd sourcing has many advantages, but it also has a major disadvantage. That is, it has meant a radical reduction in what James Curran (2011) calls journalism professionalism. Since the 1980s, Curran argues, the decline of investment in newspapers has contributed to a decline in investigative and high-quality journalism. This, combined with the atrophy of newspapers, has substantially weakened public scrutiny of government and commercial interests.
7. The Internet, including social media, has created new fields of vulnerability, particularly for bullying, hate speech, terrorism, surveillance and invasion of privacy. Online dating, for example, has become a space for sexual and romantic engagement, but also stalking and harassment (Lewis 2008).

CHAPTER SUMMARY

• The media may be categorised and studied in many different ways. Public health practitioners need to understand these media, including their limitations and respective operational opportunities for health promotion.

cont.

- At its most obvious, the media can be divided according to particular industries and platforms such as corporate broadcast media, narrowcast media, community media and interactive media. These differences are often related to the scale and means of production, distribution and consumption.

- These different media, however, often overlap. Broadcasters, for example, are increasingly using interactive media platforms to deliver their information and stories, to invite comment from users and to encourage sharing of content with niche audiences and widely dispersed social networks.

- Another important category of media refers to 'uses' and 'industries'. To this end, there is a significant difference between various forms of PR, marketing and advertising activities and industries. While health promotion and public health communicators may employ similar strategies, they may find themselves engaged in social debate, or even outright opposition to these industries and their corporate clients.

- These language wars are illustrated in the ongoing battles between public health advocates and the tobacco and pharmaceutical industries as they compete for prominence in media debates around responsibility for health, prevention and health promotion.

- While all communications industries use interactive and digital media, this form of media has particular advantages for health communication practitioners when engaging with communities to find new ways of addressing health and social issues.

References

Baudrillard, J. 1998 (orig. 1970), *The Consumer Society: Myths and Structures*, trans. C. Turner, Sage, London.

Castells, M. 2009, *The Rise of the Network Society: Economy, Society and Culture*, 2nd Edition, Wiley, New York.

Curran, J. 2011, *Media and Democracy*, Routledge, London.

Curran, J., Fenton, N. and Freedman, D. 2012, *Misunderstanding the Internet*, Routledge, London.

Dutta, M. 2011, *Communicating Social Change: Structure, Culture, and Agency*, Routledge, New York.

Ebiz. 2013, '10 most popular...', *Ebizmba*. Accessed 6 May 2014 http://www.ebizmba.com/articles/news-websites.

Freeman, B. and Chapman, S. 2010, 'British American Tobacco on Facebook: Undermining article 13 of the global World Health Organization Framework Convention on Tobacco Control', *Tobacco Control*, 19 (3): e1–e9. doi:10.1136/tc.2009.032847

Hajkowski, T. 2011, *The BBC and National Identity in Britain, 1922–53*, Manchester University Press, Manchester.

Hindman, M. 2009, *The Myth of Digital Democracy*, Princeton University Press, Princeton.

Humphery, K. 2010, *Excess: Anti-consumerism in the West*, Polity, Cambridge.

Lefebvre, R. 2013, *Social Marketing and Social Change: Strategies and Tools for Improving Health, Well-being and the Environment*, Jossey-Bass, San Francisco.

Lewis, J. 2008, *Cultural Studies*, 2nd Edition, Sage, London.

Lewis, J. 2010, *Crisis in the Global Mediasphere: Desire, Displeasure and Cultural Transformation*, Palgrave, London.

Lewis, J. 2013, *Global Media Apocalypse*, Palgrave, London.

Maine, M. and Kelly, J. 2005, *The Body Myth: Adult Women and the Pressure to be Perfect*, Wiley, New York.

McChesney, R. 2013, *Digital Disconnect: How Capitalism Is Turning the Internet against Democracy*, The New Press, New York.

Miragliotta, N. and Errington, W. 2012, 'The rise and fall and rise again of public broadcasting? The case of the Australian Broadcasting Corporation', *The Australian Journal of Public Administration*, 71 (1): 55–64.

Monbiot, G. 2011, 'The need to protect the Internet from "astroturfing" grows ever more urgent', *The Guardian*, 24 February. Accessed 6 May 2014 http://www.guardian.co.uk/environment/georgemonbiot/2011/feb/23/need-to-protect-internet-from-astroturfing.

Moynihan, R. and Cassells, A. 2005, *Selling Sickness: How the World's Biggest Drug Companies Are Turning Us All into Patients*, Allen & Unwin, Crows Nest.

Moynihan, R., Doust, J. and Henry, D. 2012, 'Preventing overdiagnosis: How to stop harming the healthy', *British Medical Journal*, 344: e3502. doi: 10.1136/bmj.e3502.

Moynihan, R. and Mintzes, B. 2010, *Sex, Lies and Pharmaceuticals: How Drug Companies Are Bankrolling the Next Big Condition for Women*, Allen & Unwin, Crows Nest.

Pullen, C. and Cooper, M. (eds) 2010, *LGBT Identity and Online New Media*, New York, Routledge.

Rheingold, H. 1993, *The Virtual Community: Homesteading on the Electronic Frontier*, Addison Wesley Publishing, Reading, MA.

Solomon, G. and Schrum, L. 2007, *Web 2.0: New Tools New Schools*, International Society for Technology in Education, Washington.

Stauber, J. 2002, *Toxic Sludge is Good For You: Lies, Damn Lies and the Public Relations Industry*, Common Courage Press, Monroe, ME.

Stoff, R. 2008, 'Astroturf roots campaign', *St Louis Journalism Review*, 1 December.

Tobacco Tactics 2011, 'Astroturfing', *Tobacco Tactics*. http://tobaccotactics.org/index.php?title=Astroturfing

Turkle, S. 1997, *Life on the Screen: Identity in the Age of the Internet*, Simon and Schuster, New York.

Turkle, S. 2011, *Alone Together: Why We Expect More from Technology and Less from Each Other*, Basic Books, New York.

Wolf, N. 1991, *The Beauty Myth: How Images of Beauty Are Used against Women*, Vintage, London.

PART II

Communicating for Health and Social Change

Social Marketing: Persuasive Communication

5

Chapter overview

This chapter provides an introduction to social marketing and its use in a wide range of public health campaigns around the world. The chapter begins with a brief exploration of the origins of social marketing, its theoretical under-pinnings and basic principles. We discuss a range of case studies to provide practical insights and illustrate some of the challenges and lessons learned. We take an in-depth look at *Act-Belong-Commit*, a community-based campaign that promotes a proactive approach to mental health and well-being in Western Australia. We also examine the counter-marketing campaign that mobilised US youth to fight back against the marketing power of multinational tobacco companies. The chapter discusses the strengths and critiques of social marketing, and we also highlight several interesting trends and emerging issues that offer new possibilities for the field.

Understanding social marketing

The origins of social marketing

Public health has a long history of providing information aiming to change people's attitudes, beliefs and behaviours that affect health. As the health promotion movement gathered momentum during the late 1980s, there was an explosion of health-related, media information campaigns. Using various combinations of print media, TV, radio and billboards, these campaigns were spectacularly effective at reaching a vast proportion of the population. Campaign evaluations showed they were effective at raising awareness about health issues and changing beliefs about risks, but that people's behaviours were much harder to change (Baum 2008).

Acknowledgement of their limited impact gave rise to calls for more expert design and development of campaigns based on claims that: 'Mass media campaigns to promote health do work. Their effectiveness, however, depends on the level of skill, experience and judgment that can be put into them' (Egger et al. 1993). Social marketing became the new buzzword as public health agencies began to work more closely with commercial advertising and marketing experts. Using models and theories derived from a combination of psychology and commercial marketing, social marketing enabled health promoters to develop more targeted and effective media campaigns.

How is social marketing used in health promotion?

Social marketing campaigns have been integral to health promotion programmes across the world, successfully contributing to reductions in death and disability from tobacco, alcohol, road trauma and a range of diseases and risk factors (Donovan & Henley 2010). In developing countries and remote communities, social marketing is widely used to increase the reach and effectiveness of traditional health information and education approaches. Recent examples include promoting hand-washing and hygiene among Australian Aboriginal communities (McDonald et al. 2011); preventing tuberculosis in Peru, diarrhoea in Madagascar and malaria in Nigeria (Cheng, Kotler & Lee 2011); and contraception and the use of condoms in a wide range of countries (Sweat et al. 2012). This approach has also been used effectively to influence social norms around gender and the treatment of women, domestic violence, child labour and unsafe agricultural practices (Donovan & Henley 2010).

Social marketing is used by a range of public health agencies, from large organisations to small, community health services. Some campaigns, such as the spectacularly effective US 'truth' campaign to reduce youth smoking, have extended over a ten-year period with funding between US$35 million and US$90 million per year (Lee 2011). Others have successfully used the principles of social marketing to inform planning for more modest, low-cost, local initiatives in small, remote communities (McDonald et al. 2011).

Definitions of social marketing vary, but they are generally developed from Andreason (1995) who describes social marketing as a process which involves

> the application of commercial marketing technologies to the analysis, planning, execution and evaluation of programs designed to influence the voluntary behaviour of target audiences in order to improve their welfare and that of society.

The essential difference between social marketing and commercial marketing is that it involves the application of marketing concepts tools and techniques to achieve socially desirable goals. That is, the outcomes are focused around the 'social common good' rather than around producing commercial rewards for the organisations engaged in marketing their products and services.

How does social marketing work?

Social marketing works by using a combination of media and interpersonal strategies to influence the knowledge, attitudes, beliefs and ultimately the behaviours of particular target groups or 'audiences'. This approach is often described as 'persuasive' communication because it moves beyond traditional health information and education, deploying sophisticated strategies designed to motivate and persuade individuals to take action.

Social marketing is generally not considered to be a population-wide health promotion approach. While some social marketing campaigns (e.g. drink driving, quit smoking) do reach a vast proportion of the population, their messages are usually designed to target particular audiences (e.g. youth drivers, smokers and their families). According to Noar (2012: 482), 'a campaign that is designed for everyone will be successful with virtually no-one'. Instead, social marketing is aimed at specific 'market segments'. During campaign development, extensive audience research is undertaken to understand the values, interests and motivations within the specific audience group as well as the likely barriers and enablers to change. The 5P's of marketing are then used to tailor the media, messages and strategies specifically to each of the audience segments they are seeking to influence. That is, having the right *product,* at the right *price,* put in the right *place,* backed by the right *promotion* and with support from the right *people* (Cheng et al. 2011; Donovan & Henley 2010).

Strengths, limitations and evidence of effectiveness
The primary focus of social marketing is to influence individual-level behaviour change. To this extent it is a midstream, rather than upstream, health promotion intervention (Keleher 2011). Research has demonstrated that social marketing campaigns can be effective for:

- raising awareness;
- increasing knowledge;
- prompting people to seek information and services;
- changing attitudes, beliefs and intentions to change behaviour; and
- achieving some changes in behaviour.

However, once the campaign has ended, these effects tend to be only short-lived unless they are supported by other, multi-level intervention strategies over the longer term (Abroms & Maibach 2008). Such strategies can include changes to policies and legislation; creating more supportive environments in workplaces, schools and families and engaging communities themselves in generating their own solutions at a local level. As we discuss later in this chapter, recent literature argues that social marketing may also have a role in contributing to these collective changes by targeting decision-makers in communities, organisations and/or governments (Donovan 2011).

Social marketing is therefore most effective when used as one strategy within a comprehensive, integrated, multi-level mix of health promotion interventions. Social marketing campaigns are usually of a limited timeframe and scope, within a wider, longer term programme. While most commonly used in the early stages of a programme, campaigns are often developed in distinct phases to be rolled out at several key stages. According to Sallis and

Owen (1998), social marketing complements other health promotion strategies through its function as:

- Educator: to introduce new ideas;
- Supporter: to reinforce old messages or maintain change;
- Promoter: to attract attention to existing programmes;
- Supplement: to community-based interventions.

Social marketing: Principles and practice

Key principles

Social marketing is different from other health promotion strategies because interventions integrate key marketing principles. The US Centers for Disease Control and Prevention (2008) identify six key marketing principles that underpin effective social marketing practice. These are summarised in Table 5.1.

Audience orientation

Successful social marketing is oriented around the interests and needs of the audience. Extensive audience research is needed to understand the values, interests and motivations within the specific audience group as well as the likely barriers and enablers to change. Understanding the ways they currently use various media helps to establish which media, channels, messages and approaches are likely to be the most effective.

While much can be learned from existing research about a target audience, most social marketing campaigns also conduct original research (surveys, focus groups, interviews) to really get to know what this audience thinks and has to say. Importantly, this research creates valuable opportunities for engaging audience members in the campaign, including development of key messages and materials and pre-testing them with their peers. Audience research is sometimes rushed or overlooked because it consumes time and resources but it is the key to ensuring that the campaign can reach and communicate effectively with its intended audience (McDonald et al. 2011).

Audience segmentation

Social marketing is aimed at specific 'market segments'. According to Noar (2012), segmentation involves a process of dividing a population into groups whose members are more similar to one another than members of other groups. Selecting a more homogenous sub-group makes it easier to tailor

Table 5.1   Six key social marketing principles

1. Audience orientation	4. Competition
2. Audience segmentation	5. Exchange (costs & benefits)
3. Focus on behaviour	6. Marketing mix

the media, messages and strategies so they resonate with this audience. Each audience 'segment' is likely to require a different approach, so it is useful to begin by developing a profile of the characteristics of each group.

Selection of audience segments can be based on factors such as demographics (age, gender, occupation, ethnic/cultural group); epidemiological data (groups who are more 'at-risk'); current behaviours (people already engaging in risky behaviour choices); and stage of readiness to change (i.e. not considering change, contemplating change, ready to try, already tried). One set of criteria for deciding which 'segments' will be the focus of the campaign is as legitimate as another but the final decisions should be based on (i) evidence and (ii) the priorities and resources of the organisation. This will enable you to develop a clear rationale for selecting each of the audience groups.

Typically, most campaigns will identify a *primary audience*: the group whose behaviour the campaign is seeking to change, and a *secondary audience*: the group/s likely to influence the primary audience (either by helping or hindering its adoption). The CDC (2008) provides an extensive list of questions to help decide on the audiences for a social marketing intervention. We provide a short version below:

Is the *primary* audience one that:

1. Is affected by the issue or risk factors for it?
2. Your partners/stakeholders most care about reaching?
3. Easily accessible by you or your partners?
4. One that fits in with your organisation's priorities?
5. Have behaviours that are easy to change?
6. Likely and willing to change their behaviour?
7. Has available existing research about them that you can use?
8. Is *not* currently being targeted with other programmes?

Is the *secondary* audience one:

1. Likely to facilitate adoption of the change?
2. Likely to inhibit change?
3. With the capacity to influence environments to make change easier and more sustained (e.g. workplaces, schools, clubs and community)?

Focus on behaviour
Social marketing aims to persuade the target audience to adopt a new behaviour, stop or reduce a current behaviour, or avoid starting a new one. The campaign should state specific behavioural goals; that is, a clear message about what behaviour is being recommended. Because behaviour change usually happens gradually, in a series of stages, this recommendation should be based on a detailed understanding of:

*   Current: what the audience is currently doing;
*   Recommended: what is the recommended behaviour;

- Possible: what small changes might be realistically possible;
- Influencers: what (or who) influences their behaviour.

According to The Health Communication Unit (THCU) (2004), the campaign should present a carefully designed message, tailored for each audience, that is based on the following three elements: What? So what? Now What? These are outlined in Table 5.2.

For example, a Canadian campaign to promote infant health by reducing women's alcohol consumption during pregnancy developed the following messages based on these elements: WHAT? Be Safe: have an alcohol-free pregnancy. SO WHAT? Drinking alcohol during pregnancy can cause birth defects and brain damage in your baby. NOW WHAT? The safest choice in pregnancy is no alcohol at all. Help is available. Talk to your healthcare provider or contact this number (THCU 2004).

Competition
Social marketing, like any form of communication, never operates in isolation from many other competing ideas and influences. Social marketing seeks to analyse the forces and other behaviours that compete against the one being recommended. Strategies are then developed to remove or minimise the appeal of the competition (Andreason 1995). For example, many social marketing campaigns focused on childhood nutrition promote the consumption of fruit as a healthy snack. The competition is a vast array of non-nutritious, processed snack foods that offer convenience, low price, good taste and fun. In order to compete, the message must emphasise the ways fresh fruit can satisfy these same needs or introduce new 'benefits' (Egger et al. 2005).

Donovan and Henley (2010) emphasise that 'competition' can also include the people, products, places and policies that work against change. For example, campaigns focused on smoking cessation have increasingly focused on the competition, the tobacco industry, with messages that undermine their credibility as good corporate citizens.

Exchange (costs and benefits)
Health promotion has a reputation for constantly trying to get people to do less of the things they enjoy (e.g. eating chocolate, smoking, watching TV) and more of the things they don't (e.g. healthy eating, drink more water, regular exercise). Social marketing uses the principle of exchange to persuade people that it's worth substituting their current behaviour choices for the alternative

Table 5.2 Message elements

WHAT?	What behaviour is recommended?
SO WHAT?	Why does it matter?
	How we, or those we care about, will benefit from this change.
NOW WHAT?	What action can we take?
	Small, easily attained steps to get started.
	Ideas that minimise the 'costs' or 'barriers' and make change easier.

behaviour being promoted in the campaign. It does this by offering people something they value in exchange for making this change.

Social marketers therefore need to understand what 'needs' are being satisfied by the current choice or behaviour. In order to compete, the new behaviour has to meet those needs, provide the same benefits or introduce new ones. This could include pleasure, risk, excitement, identity and resistance to authority (Lee 2011).

People will always weigh up the costs and benefits of making a change – so it is important to understand what the audience values and their perceptions of what they have to give up in order to get the proposed benefits. The aim of social marketing is to increase the perceived benefits of the target behaviour and minimise perceptions of its costs and barriers. The audience research should develop a detailed description of what the audience sees as the most important 'barriers, benefits and competition' for changing their behaviour.

The marketing mix

The marketing mix refers to the '5Ps' of marketing that are commonly used to ensure that the campaign is offering something of perceived value to the target audience (Donovan & Henley 2010). A typical social marketing plan will briefly describe how the campaign will address each of these elements. They are briefly explained below:

- **Product:** the targeted behaviour and its benefits. The behaviour is the 'actual' product. The promised benefits are the 'core' product.
- **Price:** what the audience gives up (the costs and the barriers and how they can be overcome); price strategies may include reducing the time and effort costs by making the 'product' more easy to do, easy to trial, widely available, easy to access or pay for.
- **Place:** where the audience gathers to 'do' the behaviour, trial it or find out about it (and how this is being made easier).
- **Promotion:** branding and project identity; communication and media strategies (the messages, media channels, methods and strategies designed specifically to reach and communicate effectively with the target audiences)
- **People and partnerships:** what services and facilities are available (trained staff and volunteers ready to assist; partnerships between local services, community groups and businesses).

Luca and Suggs (2010) add a sixth 'P' to include the following:

- **Policies:** what policies in clubs, organisations, workplaces, government support the campaign (or could change to be more supportive).

Breaking the silence on Hepatitis B in China: The 6P's in action
A recent campaign in China to reduce discrimination against people with Hepatitis B and promote strategies for preventing Hepatitis B targeted university students and people who were Hep B carriers. The general public was

the secondary audience. The *Love your Liver: Improve your Health* campaign (Cheng, Qiao & Zang 2011) addressed the 6P's as follows (Table 5.3):

Table 5.3   The 6P's in action: Hepatitis B in China

Product	Core product: A healthy liver makes you and your loved ones healthy and happy. Actual product: Protected sex using condoms. Hep B vaccinations, especially for children. Urge family and friends who are carriers to seek medical assistance.
Price	Costs: The effort to maintain healthy lifestyles. Hep B vaccinations are free for children. Vaccination is cheap for adults at only US$3. Only three shots are needed for lifetime protection.
Place	Campaign was launched in the high-profile People's Great Hall in Beijing. Hep B information made widely available. Outreach to rural areas provided extensive free vaccinations in schools and information for parents.
Promotion	Advertising, publicity (news and current affairs), special events. Student poster contests. Celebrity ambassadors who were HBV carriers. Hong Kong pop singer and HBV carrier, Andy Lau, composed a song in support of the campaign; publicly criticised schools refusing to enrol HBV carriers; and attracted widespread media and public attention to the campaign.
Partnerships	Training and resources for local health services, government health departments, universities and media outlets.
Policies	A major pharmaceutical company, already sponsoring similar campaigns in China, committed a further US$200,000 for two years extension of the campaign.

Critiques, debates and challenges for social marketing

Despite its popularity in public health, social marketing has been subject to considerable critique regarding the high costs involved, uncertain cost-effectiveness and the relatively short-term effects (Lefebvre 2013). Several other challenges for social marketing are briefly discussed below including individualism, victim blaming, inequity, expert dominance and the ethics of persuasion.

According to Keleher (2011), conventional social marketing is not consistent with the ecological model of health because of its dominant focus on individuals and their behaviour rather than the wider social, economic, environmental factors that shape people's behaviour choices. This can lead to victim blaming and moral judgements about those who do not follow the messages of health promotion campaigns. The common marketing assumption that audiences are 'free to choose' overlooks social inequities and the ways in which disadvantage restricts people's choices. Like most behaviour-focused communication, social marketing does little to challenge social structures to address inequities (Dutta 2011).

While conventional social marketing claims to be audience-oriented, it is essentially a top-down approach. Most social marketing is focused primarily on issues identified by health experts or government health authorities, and it is based around these priorities rather than issues and needs identified by communities themselves. Critics claim this reinforces the dominance of 'experts' rather than facilitating participatory and empowering approaches to problem-solving and social change (Baum 2008). Concerns are also expressed about the ethics of persuasion, whereby persuasive marketing interventions are imposed on audiences, without their consent, in order to create 'demand' based on the assumption that health-related advice, services and products are something people need and want. Furthermore, health behaviours are emphasised over other, more pressing priorities in people's lives, such as access to work, affordable food, secure housing and networks of social support (L'Etang 2008). Other critiques cast doubt on the ethics of marketing's approach to segmenting and 'profiling' audience groups in ways that foster stereotyping, ageism, racism and sexism. This is particularly the case with groups that are labelled as 'hard to reach' or 'hard to influence', such as people with low literacy, or those who are unemployed, LGBTI, living with a disability or in other minority and marginalised communities.

Addressing the critics: New and emerging approaches to social marketing

Over the last decade, new approaches to social marketing have been gradually evolving in response to these challenges and critiques. While much social marketing continues to focus on change at the level of individual behaviour, those at the cutting edge of the discipline are also exploring the possibilities for generating change at the level of communities, organisations, and environments (Lefebvre 2013; Abroms & Maibach 2008). These new approaches blend marketing models with the ecological model of health and the values and principles of health promotion. Several of these emerging perspectives are now explored in the last sections of this chapter:

- Community-based social marketing
- Ecological social marketing
- Counter-marketing
- Digital media and social marketing.

Community-based social marketing

By incorporating community development components, social marketing campaigns can substantially enhance their reach and sustainability (Donovan & Henley 2010; Bryant et al. 2007). According to the 'Community-Based Prevention Marketing' model (Bryant et al. 2007), communities should be at the centre of social marketing. In contrast to traditional 'expert led' social marketing, strategies should

- involve people in the social marketing process;
- share control over direction of the programme;

- tap into local knowledge;
- involve community members in generating ideas; and
- build partnerships and gather the community support necessary for putting ideas into action at a local level.

We now turn to a recent case study to provide practical insights and illustrate some of the challenges and lessons learned in community-based campaigns.

Act-Belong-Commit for mental health

Mentally Healthy WA's *Act-Belong-Commit* mental health promotion campaign combines social marketing with a community development approach (Donovan & Henley 2010). The overall goal of *Act-Belong-Commit* is to improve mental health and to position mental health as a whole of community issue, not just an issue for the health system. *Act-Belong-Commit* encourages individuals to be proactive in looking after their own mental health and well-being through participation in activities that enhance mental health. Based on published evidence and extensive formative research, the campaign provides a simple, three-part framework for the main campaign message:

- **Act:** Keep physically, cognitively, spiritually and socially active.
- **Belong:** Join a group, club or organisation, join in community events.
- **Commit:** Challenge yourself, learn new skills; volunteer, help others.

Following the *Act-Belong-Commit* message (Figure 5.1) can involve taking action to read a book (*Act*), join a book club (*Belong*) or volunteer for a weekly roster to listen to young children practise their reading at a local school (*Commit*).

Campaign overview

Using an ecological model, this campaign focuses on both 'people and places'. It aims to change behaviour of individual community members and also the individuals in community organisations who could influence 'places', such as clubs, community groups, public spaces and workplaces. The emphasis is on creating more supportive environments that are more welcoming for others to join up or become involved, thereby making it easier for them to follow the *Act-Belong-Commit* message.

Audiences
There are two primary audiences for the campaign: (i) Individual community members, and (ii) community groups and organisations that offered activities conducive to good mental health (e.g. libraries, sports clubs, community houses, volunteer groups, schools).

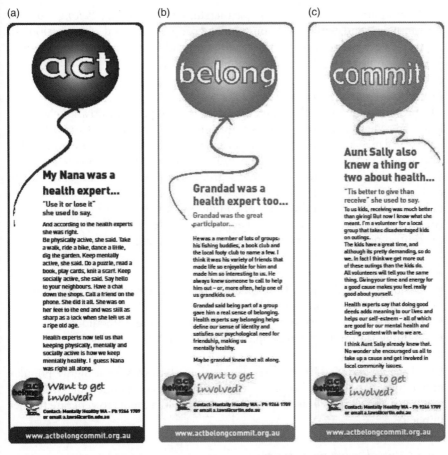

Figure 5.1   Original advertisements promoting the *Act-Belong-Commit* message

Source: *Act-Belong-Commit*

Objectives
Communication objectives are to:

- Increase awareness and understanding of mental health, encourage people to think proactively about protecting their mental health and increase awareness of activities that would help them to enhance their mental health.
- Shift community attitudes to mental health away from 'mental illness' and towards the concept of 'positive mental health'.

Behavioural objectives for the two audience groups are the following:

- Individuals: to increase participation in individual and community activities that strengthen mental health.

- Community groups: to form partnerships with the *Act-Belong-Commit* campaign and with other community groups, clubs and organisations to facilitate participation in their activities and to promote their activities under a mental health banner.

Promotional mix components

The promotional mix included media advertising in print, radio and television, radio interviews and press reports to promote the *Act-Belong-Commit* brand and its key message. Examples of the original print advertisements are provided in Figure 5.1. Merchandise, signage and logo placement were made available for use by all participating community groups. Branding of community events and activities was used to raise awareness of the *Act-Belong-Commit* messages and to strengthen the sense of community involvement in the campaign. An interactive website, linked to Facebook, Twitter and YouTube, provided the central point for community engagement, including:

- news and opportunities;
- resources for download (booklets, posters, a smartphone app, mental health facts sheets in several languages);
- merchandise (stickers, hats, bookmarks, fridge magnets); and
- communication between people and community groups.

Social media and You Tube were also used as platforms for a highly popular online 'Create your own Poster/Video' competition and online gallery. Award-winning artworks and videos were the focus of media events to generate further publicity.

Community development strategies

These involved providing a project worker in each town to facilitate the initial stages of development:

- meetings with key community representatives and local groups to discuss ways to increase social participation within the town;
- building capacity of local agencies to become involved;
- providing opportunities for local community groups to discuss strategies for helping others to follow the *Act-Belong-Commit* message;
- fostering partnerships and linkages between community groups, building support and community cohesion.

Based around the marketing principle of exchange, communities and local groups were asked to become 'social franchises' for the *Act-Belong-Commit* campaign, displaying its logos and promoting its key messages to members and others in venues and at events. In return, *Act-Belong-Commit* offered help with organising and planning events, obtaining sponsorship and funding; *Act-Belong-Commit* resources; merchandise, publicity and media coverage of their activities.

Evaluation
Ongoing process and impact evaluations show that it has been very effective in changing people's thinking about mental health; increasing participation in activities that enhance mental health; and building strong and enduring community partnerships to support mentally healthy communities. The success of the *Act-Belong-Commit* programme helped to secure a state government funding commitment for expansion of the programme across the entire state of Western Australia. A range of organisations and community groups from around the nation joined the programme.

Key success factors
Key success factors included using community-based participatory research; providing support for local community steering committees; and working in partnerships with local organisations, community groups and volunteers to facilitate their ideas for implementing *Act-Belong-Commit* in their own communities (Donovan & Henley 2010). To find out more, go to www. actbelongcommit.org.au.

Ecological social marketing: Changing people and places

Over the last decade, the role of social marketing has been revisited in relation to its potential for generating the more 'upstream' social, political and environmental changes needed to advance public health. According to Donovan (2011), social marketing needs to move beyond its traditional focus on individual voluntary behaviour change to explore its potential for influencing the environmental and commercial factors that shape people's health behaviours. He suggests that the 'new' 4P's of marketing could include the following:

- **People:** Individuals who might influence behaviour of other: as natural helpers (e.g. family, friends, people others turn to for advice), through caring roles (e.g. teachers, carers), positions of responsibility (e.g. employers), or as sources of community influence (e.g. community opinion leaders, religious leaders and popular cultural identities such as sportspeople, artists, musicians and other performers).
- **Products:** Individuals with the power to influence markets and/or the design, manufacture or marketing of *products* harmful to health, such as tobacco, processed foods, high alcohol drinks. They could also facilitate availability of less costly, more accessible and attractive, health-promoting alternatives.
- **Places:** Individuals with the power to make changes or regulate activities in *places* where people live, work and play. For example, work sites, schools, recreation areas, hospitals and sporting venues.
- **Policies:** Individuals with the *political power* to shift the allocation of resources to increase equity of access and opportunities in society. For example, government representatives, legal practitioners, education and health services.

Donovan proposes a more 'ecological' approach that targets 'gatekeepers' and decision-makers in communities and organisations with the capacity to influence the people, places, products and policies that impact on health. Within this approach, social marketing is used to target individuals (to influence behaviour choices), social networks (to exchange ideas, helpful strategies and support for behaviour change) and decision-makers (to influence organisations and environments so they are more conducive to healthy behaviour choices).

Counter-marketing: Using opponents' marketing tactics for a good cause

The principles of marketing are also used in health promotion to oppose industries and corporations with vested interests in health-damaging products and behaviours such as the alcohol, tobacco, processed foods, firearms and advertising industries. Counter-marketing involves health promotion advocates using their knowledge of marketing principles to identify and monitor industry marketing tactics and develop appropriate 'counter-marketing' strategies (Egger et al. 2005).

Counter-marketing has been used as an activist tactic for health promotion since the 1970s, although it was often referred to as 'subvertising'. Early examples include Australia's *BUGA-UP*, a group of health activists who took disruptive action to get people's attention, influence public opinion and stimulate debate about the pervasive influence of unhealthy advertising:

> [T]obacco and other advertising was everywhere – indoors, outdoors, in cinemas and on television . . . Huge tobacco advertisements covered the sides of buildings, or blared from their rooftops. Freeways and roads had tobacco signs along the way. Billboards were at railway stations and between stops, in train carriages and on buses.
>
> (Buga-Up n.d.)

Creating their own 'brand', BUGA-UP (Billboard Utilising Graffitists Against Unhealthy Promotions) embarked on a coordinated campaign that involved 're-facing' outdoor tobacco advertising. BUGA-UP members scaled huge billboards to cover the ads with anti-tobacco graffiti designed to 'name and shame' tobacco companies. Messages were unequivocally about blame and responsibility: 'Show your face, drug pusher!', 'Death sentence!', 'Killers'. The graffitists also ridiculed and defaced images of celebrities who had received huge payments to advertise cigarettes. Others manipulated the wording of advertising slogans to force viewers' attention onto less well-recognised health risks: 'Smoking stinks mate!', 'Tobacco give you smokers droop . . .'. Slogans such as 'Anyhow, have a Winfield!' became 'So many women hate Winfield fools!' (see BUGAUP Catalogue 1981, at http://www.bugaup.org).

While more conservative public health organisations distanced themselves from BUGA-UP's approach, their disruptive action gained substantial publicity. Their controversial 'Robin Hood' tactics had an important agenda-setting role in shifting blame away from millions of individual smokers and onto a small group of powerful, multinational tobacco companies. This helped to foster public support, from both smokers and non-smokers, for the gradual introduction of comprehensive tobacco control initiatives over the years that followed (Chapman 2007, 1996). To see photos of a wide range of BUGA UP activist's billboard graffiti, and learn more about their work, go to http://www.bugaup.org

The truth campaign

More recently in the United Kingdom, the United States and Australia, counter-marketing has been used effectively to compete against tobacco industry tactics using an integrated combination of advertising, public relations, media advocacy, grassroots marketing and media literacy (ASH Scotland 2013; Chapman 2007; CDC 2003). For example, the US *truth* counter-marketing campaign has contributed to sustained reductions in youth smoking by mobilising young people against the tobacco industry. The campaign engages youth in collective action to undermine the reputation of big tobacco companies, portraying them as greedy and dishonest (hence the '*truth*' brand). The campaign aimed to expose corporate greed, unethical marketing tactics, lack of responsibility and massive profiteering from persuading young people to start and become addicted to smoking (Allen et al. 2009; CDC 2003). The aims of *truth* were to reduce youth smoking by getting young people to see that big tobacco companies are trying to manipulate them.

Background to the issue

Teenagers' resistance to anti-smoking campaigns is well known and, in tobacco control circles, youth are still considered one of the hardest to reach groups (Allen et al. 2009). For many teens, smoking has meanings around independent identity, risk-taking and resistance to authority. Many studies show that teenage smokers reject the meanings carried in expert public health warnings about negative health effects and long-term health risks. For decades, anti-smoking campaigns that focused on individual behaviour-change had very little impact on youth. Furthermore, huge multi-national tobacco corporations, such as Philip Morris, have funded their own social marketing campaigns like 'Think. Don't Smoke'. The campaign had no success in reducing youth smoking but, not surprisingly, it resulted in more *positive* youth attitudes towards the tobacco industry itself (Farrelly et al. 2002). The ineffective Philip Morris campaign was little more than a public relations exercise – a tactic used by the company to create an impression of their 'corporate social responsibility' (see chapters 9 and 10).

Truth campaign overview: Aims, objectives and audiences

In contrast, the Florida-based *truth* campaign has provided an alternative approach that taps into youth cultures and resistance to authority. Since 1998, the *truth* campaign has sought to break the hold of tobacco industry advertising over youth audiences by exposing Big Tobacco's deceptive marketing and manufacturing practices. When a leading tobacco company launched legal action against the campaign, from 2001 until 2006, this only served to strengthen the resolve of youth coalitions to continue the fight. Awareness and support for *truth* continued to grow. The campaign has been extremely effective across all measures of attitudes and actual smoking behaviour among young people as well as the wider population (Lee 2011; Allen et al. 2009).

Audiences

The *primary audience* was teenagers aged 12–17 because nearly 80% of smokers begin in this age group. The *secondary audience* was young people aged 18–24 because formative research showed this group is an important influence on teenagers and they are often asked to give, or sell, cigarettes to teens.

Objectives

Communication objectives were to (i) increase youth awareness of the effects, social cost and addictiveness of smoking and the tactics used by the tobacco industry to target them and (ii) change beliefs from seeing smoking as an expression of independence to understanding that smoking is no longer 'the norm' for youth and that they are in control and empowered to make a choice. Behavioural objectives were for youth to express their concerns about the tactics and lies of the tobacco industry and share these with other young people. Importantly, the campaign did not tell young people 'not' to smoke.

Promotion strategies: Media and communication

Like the marketing tactics of big tobacco companies, the *truth* campaign taps into youth culture and has placed particular emphasis on peer-to-peer promotion and interactive media. The campaign is promoted through grassroots advocacy and a youth-driven advertising campaign. Campaign materials use gritty imagery, video and urban streetscapes with youth delivering their own hard-hitting version of 'the facts' along with a call to action. The campaign has effectively shifted the focus of the 'problem' from youth to the tobacco industry. In a neat inversion of conventional victim-blaming, this campaign suggests to young people that 'You aren't the problem. They are'.

Promotional strategies included the following:

- advertising in entertainment venues;
- interactive websites (with polls related to facts about tobacco and tobacco companies, embedded videos, screensavers and downloadable items);
- merchandise give-aways (hats, T-shirts and wallets created by youth designers);
- grassroots outreach trucks at popular events and festivals with DJs, video monitors and a youth 'crew' spreading the word about *truth* and how to get involved;
- tour stops with *truth* crews holding dance contests, freestyle rap battles and DJ lessons;

- *truth* homepages on popular social networking sites linking back to the main website where teens can meet crew members, follow their blogs, get event updates and free tickets;
- creating online communities through social media and linking them with advocacy and activist groups focused around a common cause (Lee 2011).

The *truth* campaign illustrates a shift in social marketing approaches from traditional, expert-led communication 'telling people what they should do' towards a more contemporary cultural studies approach where audiences are active participants in the communication process, sharing information and ideas, creating networks for action and generating their own strategies for mobilising others. The truth campaign engages with youth culture, with young people playing a key role in designing all aspects of the programme and materials. By tapping into what motivates teenagers around independent identity, risk-taking and resistance to authority, *truth* has created opportunities for youth to recognise they have a powerful collective voice against the tobacco industry and a legitimate role in activism for social change.

Note: All campaign tactics, resources, activities and interactive media for each phase of the campaign are available at *www.thetruth.com* and www. protectthetruth.org. Lessons learned from this campaign have also been compiled in a guide to counter-marketing, 'Designing and Implementing an Effective Tobacco Counter-Marketing Campaign' (CDC 2003).

Social media in social marketing

The Internet and interactive digital media are fundamental tools of all marketing, including social marketing. Mobile and social media, in particular, are enabling radical shifts in the ways social marketing is practised (Lefebvre 2013). In this last section, we discuss some of their strengths and limitations and we provide practical insights for using interactive, networked media in social marketing.

Campaign websites

A campaign website is the most basic digital media communication tool for a social marketing campaign. Typically, this will be linked to the organisation hosting (or funding) the campaign and so the features of the website will depend on the available resources and media policies of the organisation overseeing the campaign. It is important to work closely with the organisation's media team to ensure the online presence consistently uses the 'branding' elements of the campaign (logos, colour-schemes, sponsors). This also applies to all partner organisations involved in the campaign.

Even for people working on a small, local campaign, the wide availability of open-source software for developing a basic site means that even small-scale campaigns can build an online presence. The advantages of a traditional, one-way website are that the 'experts' can maintain control of content (information, key messages, public relations); however, a non-interactive website has limited capacity to foster community engagement with the campaign.

Using interactive digital media

Social media can enable a campaign to reach large audiences, including online communities of thousands of people, with a single click, very quickly, and at very low cost. Social media are also extremely effective at tapping into smaller, niche audiences through networks of people with similar interests and social connections. In both cases, interactive media create opportunities for encouraging participation, conversation and community around the issues in the campaign (CDC 2012a).

Web 2.0 technologies have enabled blogs, wikis, file-sharing and social networking sites (such as Facebook, Twitter, YouTube, Flickr) to:

- increase campaign awareness and credibility;
- build relationships with key audiences;
- use comments, reposting and sharing to engage new audiences;
- create opportunities for users to generate some of the site's content.

Video, games, buttons, widgets, text and multi-media messaging and other interactive media tools also provide a variety of ways of engaging traditionally 'hard to reach' audiences with campaign issues and content, as well as creating new content for themselves and sharing it with others (see Parvanta et al. 2011).

When using a website with interactive features or links to social media, it needs to be appropriately hosted, monitored regularly, and administration should follow recommended ethical and best practice guidelines. Seeman (2008) provides useful insights for addressing important ethical issues, such as confidentiality, use of personal information, accessibility, accountability, transparency of authorship and sponsorship.

Two excellent practical guides to planning and using social media can be found in the 'The Health Communicator's Social Media Toolkit' (CDC 2011) and 'Writing for social media' (CDC 2012a). Several interesting discussions about practical strategies, ethics and the use of social media in marketing for public health can be found in Thackeray et al. (2012) and Neiger et al. (2012).

Viral and buzz marketing

The use of Web 2.0 technologies for persuasive communication in social marketing is not without its challenges. Recent public health interventions have experimented with several social media strategies commonly used in commercial marketing in order to increase the reach and credibility of their messages with target audiences (see Parvanta & Parvanta 2011: 231–233). These include the following:

- viral marketing: encouraging individuals to 'share' compelling information, and
- buzz marketing: selecting individuals from within existing online communities to become 'buzz agents' who are not identified as being on the marketing team but who strategically post content to create a 'buzz' around the issue and associated services or products.

While these are powerful marketing strategies, they also raise important ethical questions about the extent to which 'social marketers' should mimic the tactics of commercial marketing.

For example, viral and buzz marketing through social media have also been used by big corporations, such as Phillip Morris and British American Tobacco, to get around tobacco advertising restrictions. In a controversial tactic called 'astroturfing', employees create a variety of false online personas and/or organisations who participate in social media conversations in ways that are favourable towards smoking and tobacco. They use strategies such as casually chatting about the tobacco products they like and/or generating a buzz around promotional events, music festivals and promotion parties. Astroturfers also work through a range of social networking sites to actively undermine the opinions and posts of people who challenge their activities. Strategies have ranged from providing support for existing 'smokers rights groups' to the corporate creation of false social media groups with the same intent (Laverack 2012; Tobacco Tactics 2012; Freeman & Chapman 2010).

The increasing use of viral and buzz marketing in health promotion brings a number of ethical concerns about transparency, invasion of privacy, protection from harm and denial of important consumer rights (see Monbiot 2011). Furthermore, commercial marketing practices such as astroturfing have been the subject of legal investigation and prosecution in a number of countries (New York State Office of the Attorney General 2013). These studies raise important issues about the ways in which public health marketers may also risk compromising their ethical responsibilities by invading social media spaces to achieve their marketing ends.

Social media: A new generation of social marketing?

According to Clow and Baack (2007), the last decade has seen shifts in the way marketing is conducted:

1. From one-way media advertising to multiple communication channels and technologies.
2. From mass media to more specialised (niche) media for smaller, specific target audiences.
3. From expert-dominated approach to an audience-centred approach.
4. Greater agency accountability for conducting marketing in ethical and equitable manner.
5. 24/7 Internet availability and access to information, goods and services.

Where social marketing has traditionally communicated with audiences based on traditional, linear 'source-message-channel-receiver' models, the discipline is moving towards a 'cultural model' of communication in which active audiences are engaging with texts, media-making and with each other in a dynamic and collaborative process. Rather than designing one-way messages for target audiences, social marketers are communicating about health in a world where audiences 'expect to talk back to us, and with each other' (Lefebvre 2013).

Audience groups are becoming smaller as they select media content to suit their tastes and preferences. Web 2.0 technologies are enabling people to collaborate and share information as they interact, create new content and share it with others of similar interests and social connections. This has stimulated considerable rethinking of the 'Ps' of marketing to make the most of its potential for interactivity, networking and participation. Lefebvre (2013) proposes 5E's of social marketing where the aim is to educate, entertain, enable and empower people to become evangelists for social and cultural change. He describes the new social marketing as being essentially about community. It involves a network of 'conversations' with multiple opportunities for people to participate, exchange ideas, create content and share.

According to Lefebvre (2013), social and mobile technologies are creating new opportunities for social marketing to move away from 'messages and target audiences' to become more involved in:

- Enhancing existing linkages between people and communities, not only to share knowledge and resources but also to deepen and strengthen support between people trying to make positive, prosocial change;
- Nurturing and sustaining new types of linkages that bring people together (around similar interests, a shared 'mission', communities addressing a common problem);
- Better engaging communities in problem-solving by creating new networks of people supporting community-level change;
- Weaving together existing networks of groups not normally accustomed to working together to create new sources of inspiration and power to address health and social issues;
- Engage communities in new ways to mobilise and to engage with public health priorities.

However, Lefebvre (2013) argues that this potential can only be realised if experts are prepared to relinquish some of their control over the social marketing process so it is less prescriptive, top-down and expert-led. This includes genuinely involving audiences as collaborators and co-creators with a lead role in developing strategies and implementing them. Rather than being the 'source' of communications, professionals and organisations need to see themselves as being part of a 'conversation' in which audiences are generating much of what is being communicated.

As interactive communication technologies keep evolving, people expect to be active participants and to have a voice. A vast array of communities are creating their own ways of communicating about themselves and their issues, creating stories, sharing them and opening up their perspectives to the wider global community. According to Lefebvre (2013), the implications of this are that public health communicators' 'expert' role is likely to need a radical overhaul if we are to make the most of these new technologies, cultures and opportunities. With these thoughts in mind, the following chapters will go on to explore a range of participatory, community-based approaches to health communication.

CHAPTER SUMMARY

- Social marketing applies commercial marketing concepts and techniques to the design of communication strategies that aim to influence behaviour change towards socially desirable goals.

- It is effective for awareness raising, attitude and short-term behaviour change and is more sustainable if supported by community development strategies.

- New 'ecological' approach to social marketing is focused on influencing individual behaviour, social networks and also decision-makers in communities and organisations with the capacity to affect upstream influences on behaviour.

- Digital technologies and interactive, social media are creating opportunities for shifting the role of audiences from being 'targets' of social marketing to being active participants, co-creators of content and collaborative drivers of the process.

- Key questions for social marketing in the networked, digital world are focused on how campaigns can:
  o Enhance existing linkages between people;
  o Help develop new types of linkages that bring people together to address common problems;
  o Identify, encourage and enable natural helpers in social networks to facilitate their role as health promoters;
  o Better engage communities in problem-solving to address health and social equity;
  o Weave together existing networks of individuals, organisations and communities to create new sources of power to address health and social issues.

References

Abroms, L. and Maibach, E. 2008, 'The effectiveness of mass communication to change public behaviour', *Annual Reviews of Public Health*, 29: 219–234.

Allen, J. A., Vallone, D., Vargyas, E. and Healton, C. G. 2009, 'The truth®campaign: Using countermarketing to reduce youth smoking', in B. Healey and R. Zimmerman (eds), *The New World of Health Promotion, New Program Development, Implementation and Evaluation*, Jones and Bartlett Learning, Sudbury, MA, 195–215.

Andreason, A. 1995, *Marketing and Social Change: Changing Behaviour to Promote Health, Social Development and the Environment*, Jossey Bass, San Francisco.

ASH Scotland 2013, Taking Action on Smoking and Health. Accessed 6 May 2014 www.ashscotland.org.uk.

Baum, F. 2008, *The New Public Health: An Australian Perspective*, 3rd Edition, Oxford, Melbourne.

Bryant, C., Brown, K., Mcdermott, R., Forthofer, M., Bumpus, E., Calkins, S. and Zapata, L. 2007, 'Community-based prevention marketing', Health Promotion Practice, 8 (2): 154–163.

BUGA UP n.d. *Billboard Utilising Graffitists against Unhealthy Promotions.* Accessed 6 May 2014 http://www.bugaup.org/publications.

Centers for Disease Control and Prevention (CDC) 2003, *Designing and Implementing an Effective Tobacco Counter-Marketing Campaign*, U.S. Department of Health and Human Services, Atlanta, GA. Accessed 6 May 2014 http://www.cdc.gov/tobacco/stateandcommunity/counter_marketing/manual/index.htm.

Centers for Disease Control and Prevention (CDC) 2008, *Social Marketing for Nutrition and Physical Activity Web Course*, Division of Nutrition, Physical Activity, and Obesity, U.S.

Chapman, S. 1996, 'Civil disobedience and tobacco control: The case of BUGA UP', *Tobacco Control*, 5 (3): 179–185.

Chapman, S. 2007, *Public Health Advocacy and Tobacco Control: Making Smoking History*, Oxford, Blackwell.

Cheng, H., Kotler, P. and Lee, N. 2011, *Social Marketing for Public Health: Global Trends and Success Stories*, Jones and Bartlett, Sudbury, MA.

Cheng, H., Qiao, J. and Zhang, H. 2011, 'Love your liver, improve your health: A Hepatitis B prevention and educational campaign in China', in H. Cheng, P. Kotler and N. Lee (eds), *Social Marketing for Public Health: Global Trends and Success Stories*, Jones and Bartlett, Sudbury, MA.

Clow, K. and Baack, D. 2007, *Integrated Advertising, Promotion, and Marketing Communications*, Pearson Education Limited, Harlow, UK.

Donovan, R. 2011, 'Ecological social marketing in public health change programs', *Australian Review of Public Affairs*, 10 (1): 23–40.

Donovan, R. and Henley, R. 2010, *Principles and Practice of Social Marketing: An International Perspective*, Cambridge University Press, Cambridge.

Dutta, M. 2011, *Communicating Social Change: Structure, Culture, and Agency*, Routledge, New York.

Egger, G., Spark, R. and Donovan, R. 1993, *Health and the Media: Principles and Practices for Health Promotion*, McGraw-Hill, Sydney, 161–173.

Egger, G., Spark, R. and Donovan, R. 2005, 'Focus on populations: Social marketing and the media', *Health Promotion Strategies and Methods*, McGraw-Hill, Sydney.

Farrelly, M., Healton, C., Davis, K., Messeri, P., Hersey, J. and Haviland, L. 2002, 'Getting to the truth: Evaluating national tobacco countermarketing campaigns', *American Journal of Public Health*, 92 (6): 901–907.

Freeman, B. and Chapman, S. 2007, 'Is "YouTube" telling or selling you something? Tobacco content on the YouTube video-sharing website', *Tobacco Control*, 16 (3): 207–210.

Freeman, B. and Chapman, S. 2010, 'British American Tobacco on Facebook: Undermining article 13 of the global World Health Organization Framework Convention on Tobacco Control', *Tobacco Control*, 19 (3): e1–e9. doi:10.1136/tc.2009.032847

Keleher, H. 2011, 'Social marketing', in H. Keleher and C. MacDougall (eds), *Understanding Health*, 3rd edition, 249–258.

Laverack, G. 2012, 'Health activism', *Health Promotion International*, 27 (4): 429–434.

L'Etang, J. 2008, *Public Relations: Concepts, Practice and Critique*, Sage, London.

Lee, N. 2011, 'Reducing tobacco use in the United States: A public health success story so far', in H. Cheng, P. Kotler and N. Lee (eds), *Social Marketing for Public Health: Global Trends and Success Stories*, Jones and Bartlett, Sudbury, MA.

Lefebvre, R. C. 2013, *Social Marketing and Social Change: Strategies and Tools for Improving Health, Well-being and the Environment*, Jossey-Bass, San Francisco.

Luca, N. and Suggs, S. 2010, 'Strategies for the social marketing mix: A systematic review, *Social Marketing Quarterly*, 16 (4): 122–149.

McDonald, E., Slavin, N., Bailie, R. and Schobben, X.2011, 'No germs on me: A social marketing campaign to promote hand-washing with soap in remote Australian aboriginal communities', *Global Health Promotion*, 18 (1): 62–65.

Monbiot, G. 2011, 'The need to protect the internet from "Astroturfing" grows ever more urgent', *The Guardian*, London, UK. Accessed 6 May 2014 http://www.theguardian.com/environment/georgemonbiot/2011/feb/23/need-to-protect-internet-from-astroturfing.

Neiger, B. L., Thackeray, R., Van Wagenen, S. A., Hanson, C. L., West, J. H., Barnes, M. D. and Fagen, M. C. 2012, 'Use of social media in health promotion: Purposes, key performance indicators, and evaluation metrics', *Health Promotion Practice*, 13 (2): 159–164.

New York State Office of the Attorney General (2013), A.G. Schneiderman Announces Agreement With 19 Companies To Stop Writing Fake Online Reviews And Pay More Than $350,000 In Fines. State of New York. Accessed 6 May 2014 http://www.ag.ny.gov/press-release/ag-schneiderman-announces-agreement-19-companies-stop-writing-fake-online-reviews-and.

Noar, S. 2012, 'An Audience-Channel-Message-Evaluation (ACME) framework for health Communication campaigns', *Health Promotion Practice*, 13 (4): 481–488.

Parvanta, C., Nelson, D. E., Parvanta, S. A. and Harner, R. N. 2011, *Essentials of Public Health Communication*, Jones and Bartlett Learning, Sudbury, MA.

Parvanta, C. and Parvanta, P. 2011, 'It's a multimedia world', in C. Parvanta, D. E. Nelson, S. A. Parvanta and R. N. Harner (eds), *Essentials of Public Health Communication*, Jones and Bartlett Learning, Sudbury, MA, 205–239.

Sallis, J. and Owen, N. 1998, *Physical Activity and Behavioural Medicine*, Sage, London.

Seeman, N. 2008, 'Inside the health blogosphere: Quality, governance and the new innovation leaders', *Healthcare Quarterly*, 12 (1): 101–108.

Sweat, M., Denison, J., Kennedy, C., Tedrow, V. and O'Reilly, K. 2012, 'Effects of condom social marketing on condom use in developing countries: A systematic review and meta-analysis, 1990–2010', *Bulletin of the World Health Organization*, 90 (8): 613–622.

Thackeray, R., Neiger, B. L. and Keller, H. 2012, 'Integrating social media and social marketing: A four-step process', *Health Promotion Practice*, 13 (2): 165–168.

The Health Communication Unit (THCU) 2004, 'Be safe have an alcohol free pregnancy, case study series 3', *The Health Communication Unit, Centre for Health Promotion*, University of Toronto, Ontario. Accessed 6 May 2014 http://www.thcu.ca.

Tobacco Tactics 2012, 'Astroturfing', *Tobacco Tactics*. Accessed 6 May 2014 http://tobaccotactics.org/index.php?title=Astroturfing.

Participatory Communication for Health: Working with Communities

6

Chapter overview

This chapter explores participatory approaches to communication for health and explains the importance of working *with* communities when communicating about health and social change. We examine the principles and practice of participatory approaches, why they are important and how they can be used in communication for health and social change. We discuss a range of case studies to provide practical insights and illustrate some of the challenges and lessons learned. We begin with an inspiring example focused on sex-worker communities in Kolkata, India. We take an in-depth look at the use of Photovoice by young people engaged in youth violence prevention in the United Kingdom and the United States. We also explore the use of participatory communication by refugees, minority ethnic communities and people with spinal cord injuries to create opportunities for engaging in dialogue and community decision-making about health.

Introduction to participatory health communication

Participatory communication refers to communication strategies that are created *for* communities *by* communities themselves. In the previous chapter, we explored the use of social marketing as a communication strategy in broadcast, mass media campaigns. These campaigns are extremely effective at reaching a large proportion of the population, including particular target audience 'segments'. However, they are consistently less successful with minority and marginalised groups, and people who do not normally access mainstream media due to poverty, low literacy, disability, cultural preferences or simply personal choice (Lemelle et al. 2011). These groups are sometimes referred to by health social marketers as 'hard-to-reach' and/or 'hard-to-influence' (Egger 2005). However, there is now a strong and growing literature with many examples that demonstrate the strengths of community-based, participatory health communication for working with diverse communities (Dutta 2011; Minkler & Wallerstein 2010; Dreher 2010; Zoller & Dutta 2008).

Participatory communication is also useful when working with groups (for example sex workers or intravenous drug users) who have quite specific health risks and/or concerns. While explicit information about particular high-risk sexual practices or safer injecting is useful for these groups, it is not always practical or possible to communicate about these issues with the general population or through mainstream media. Much of this content can be culturally (and politically) sensitive and would need to be diluted substantially for general audiences, making it relatively useless for the groups who need it most (Stanley & MacLean 2005).

Community-based, participatory communication is often the best approach for working with people who identify as being part of marginal and minority groups, for whom mainstream health communication messages are seen as irrelevant to the realities of their day-to-day lives. As Basu and Dutta (2011) note, 'identity' is of central importance for people in marginalised communities. People's sense of individual identity, community and belonging to a marginal group is expressed through their everyday practices. This includes the ways they communicate about health within their communities and also how they engage with, and express resistance to, mainstream health promotion.

Participatory health communication approaches have been used in a variety of ways with: migrant and refugee communities around young women's sexual health (Cheatham-Rojas & Shen 2010); stigmatised groups such as the transgendered community (Clements-Nolle & Bachrach 2010); sensitive issues and hidden populations such as gay men in the US military (Pullen & Cooper 2010); socially and geographically isolated communities such as people living with spinal cord injuries (Newman 2010); prisoners (Anderson 2012a); and marginalised indigenous groups with low levels of literacy (Lardeau et al. 2011).

These examples demonstrate the importance of facilitating people's participation in the *process* of health communication. Participatory health communication shared through peers with similar lifestyles and values ('people like me') is more likely to generate meaningful and sustainable change than health messages imposed on people by outsider 'experts' or public health authorities (Stanley & MacLean 2005). We now turn to a case study to illustrate the use of participatory health communication based on extensive work by Basu and Dutta (2011, 2009) with marginalised communities of sex workers.

Sex workers and HIV: 'We are mothers first'

In India, female commercial sex workers are the group at highest risk of becoming infected with HIV/AIDS and transmitting the disease to others. According to Basu and Dutta (2011), these women continue to be marginalised and stigmatised by mainstream Indian society. Discrimination is further amplified through legal systems and portrayals in news, film and academic scripts depicting them as insufficient women, incapable of caring for themselves and their children.

Commercial sex workers in the Sonagachi and Kalighat communities of Kolkata, India, have an interesting history of resistance to safe-sex messages from outside experts promoting the use of condoms. For a long time, these women have been well aware of the increased risk of contracting HIV/AIDS, but clients pay more for sex without condoms and these women are extremely poor. Most are without partners or husbands and originally started selling sex as a means of survival. Often, unprotected sex is forced upon them through coercion and/or violence. Many of these commercial sex workers (CSWers) are also mothers of young children (Basu & Dutta 2009) (Plate 6.1).

With the support of a local doctor, Samarjit Janatwo, two sex-worker-run programmes were initiated in the early 1990s: the Sonagachi HIV/AIDS Intervention Programme (SHIP) and New Light's HIV/AIDS Project. Both have highly successful in increasing the rate of condom use amongst sex workers – from 3% in 1992 to 90% in 1999. More than a decade later, both programmes continue to have long-lasting effects on the well-being of women and children in these CSWer communities (Basu & Dutta 2009).

How has this been possible? These programmes have adopted an alternative approach to traditional, expert-led behaviour-change campaigns and instead

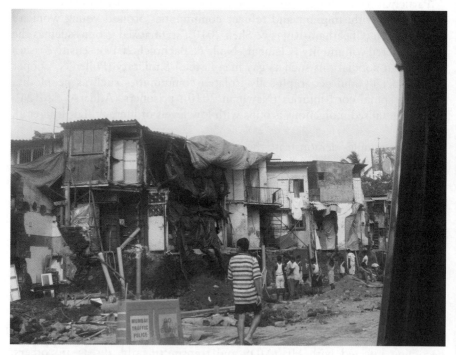

Plate 6.1   Slum communities in India (2008)

Source: Belinda Lewis

they are focused on a participatory, community-based approach. Starting with a leadership group of 12 sex workers, CSWers were encouraged and supported to strengthen the informal networks where women were already talking together, listening to each others' stories, identifying problems and collectively devising solutions.

Rather than focusing specifically on sex work, women talked together about their everyday lives. As 'mothers first', their most immediate concerns were about the safety of their children while they are working and being able to provide them with adequate food and shelter. They also wanted to ensure that their adolescent daughters could access alternatives to sex work by completing their school education. For these women, working without condoms earns more money in less time and this means more time is available for their roles and responsibilities as mothers. But paradoxically, it also increases their risk of contracting HIV/AIDS.

Through these participatory networks, CSWers decided they didn't want or need any more top-down, condom use campaigns. They wanted to find ways to address the factors in their living and working conditions that made it almost impossible for them to follow safe-sex, HIV/AIDS prevention messages. Finding ways to negotiate these more pressing priorities and personal concerns would make it easier for them to focus on their own health and reducing their risk of HIV/AIDS.

According to Basu and Dutta (2009), the 'New Light' programme has now worked collaboratively with these CSWer networks for over a decade, combining HIV/AIDS awareness and prevention with community development activities. Sex worker mothers have been active participants in all aspects of these activities, and their programme has secured funding and support to provide daily meals to more than 125 children of sex workers; five free health clinics every week; and a residential hostel for adolescent girl children of CSWers. Without having to worry about what their children are going to eat and where they will sleep, CSWers are more able to resist being coerced into unsafe sex.

The SHIP CSWer networks have also grown substantially from the original 12 women. More than 20 years later, these networks continue to advocate for sex worker rights and services so that they can more easily protect themselves and their families. Successes include community health services, stronger policing and violence prevention and recognition of their rights to be treated with fairness and respect. SHIP is now part of the Durbar collective (which means 'unstoppable' in Bengali) that represents 65,000 sex-workers (male, female and transgender) and is active in identifying and challenging the underlying socio-structural factors that help perpetuate stigma, material deprivation and social exclusion of sex-workers.

This participatory approach to health communication has fostered ownership, pride, and collective confidence in taking action towards the social change that is needed to address health issues and concerns within these communities. For more detailed information and inspiration, go to www.newlightindia.org and www.durbar.org.

What is participatory health communication?

According to Dutta (2011), health communication is more effective, empowering and equitable when it is focused around strategies created *for* communities *by* communities themselves.

This approach is based on the idea that community members already have a great deal of insider knowledge about health issues within their community and the factors that influence their experiences of health. This places them in a good position to know what health communication strategies are most likely to work. When the authority of community members is acknowledged, and they are supported in taking responsibility for communicating about health, new opportunities are created for community members themselves to facilitate change. This includes participating in ongoing dialogue with health experts and decision-makers in governments and organisations. PHC aims to build capacity and opportunities for communities to effectively communicate with each other and broader society about their community strengths, as well as the health problems facing their communities, and the strategies through which they might be addressed. Through this process, community people are enabled as citizens and as active participants in the institutions and decisions that affect their lives.

Key principles

Participatory health communication is 'culture-centered'; that is, it locates culture at the centre of the communication process and integrates the cultural practices, values, concerns and needs of the community. A participatory approach is community-driven in that it foregrounds the voices of community members and their own articulations of health problems facing their communities. It respects and emphasises the agency (ability) of community members to frame solutions and communication strategies. Consequently, the role of experts is less about telling people what they need to 'do' or change, and instead involves listening, responding to and helping people give direction to their own change.

PHC works in partnership 'with' communities rather than 'on' them. It involves facilitating people's participation by creating opportunities for social dialogue and fostering the supportive environments needed for this process to take place. Participatory approaches emphasise the *processes* in communication, including engagement, participation and empowerment. The desired outcome is empowerment *through* participation: people representing themselves, telling their own stories and putting forward their points of view.

Where experts have traditionally determined whose voices are included and how they are used to generate change, participatory health communication seeks to foreground the perspectives of community members, and particularly those whose voices might otherwise remain unheard. It seeks to create opportunities for people to communicate about their health priorities and concerns, including the social and structural influences on health in their local communities. This approach to health communication is about bringing people together and empowering them to become actively involved in generating solutions to health problems. It is also about creating opportunities to speak with, and be heard by, community leaders and decision-makers in the spaces where the decisions that affect whole communities are made (Vaughan 2010). When participatory approaches are used, community members are more likely to have a sense of ownership over both the process and the outcomes, making these more meaningful and more likely to be maintained long after any official 'intervention' has ended (Basu & Dutta 2009).

Participation

Within many health communication campaigns, it is common to involve community members as participants in formative research, pre-testing messages or being the 'messengers' for a campaign agenda. Within these approaches, community members are often treated as passive audiences rather than initiators or drivers of the programme. On the other hand, participatory approaches involve community members in actively driving the agenda for change by having a genuine role in the selection of issues, design, implementation, evaluation of strategies or programmes and determining future areas for action (Basu & Dutta 2009). PHC also recognises that minority and marginal communities are not homogenous and that strategies are needed to facilitate participation by those with less access to communicative spaces (such as children, the elderly, people with low literacy, living with disability or chronic illness). As we demonstrate in the case studies covered in the next few chapters, participatory approaches seek to foster a sense of community ownership, responsibility and pride in the communication platforms that are created and sustained by people in minority and marginalised communities (Minkler & Wallerstein 2010).

Community

When we talk about community, we are referring to groups of people who are linked in some way through what they have in common. A 'community of place' may be centred around a shared location or geographic area where people live, work or play. 'Communities of interest' may be linked by such things as shared values, ethnicity, religion, health experiences, recreational activities, sexuality or political interests. While people in the same geographic area don't necessarily share a sense of community, communities can be created and sustained across vast distances by people from different cultures and backgrounds, who are never likely to meet in person. In each case, communities are created around a sense of shared identity, and they are maintained and strengthened through social interactions (Israel et al. 2010).

As we noted in our earlier discussion of culture (see Chapter 3), most people are part of several different communities and cultures. Our sense of identity, community and belonging is complex, overlapping and at times conflicting. While the term 'community' implies a simple grouping of people, communities are actually complex social systems made up of people with diverse interests and they often involve unequal power relations. According to Taylor et al. (2008), it is important to dispense with the normative 'myth' of community as a cohesive, united group. Practitioners should also be sensitive to the different perspectives and political struggles that occur within communities.

Origins and theoretical underpinnings

Participatory approaches to community-based health communication have their origins in the theoretical perspectives of cultural studies, post-colonialism, feminism and sub-altern studies (Minkler & Wallerstein 2010; Dutta 2008). These theories have a particular focus on issues of culture and identity, marginalisation, power and resistance, and they are often deployed by scholars and practitioners who are interested in challenging socially structured inequalities.

Following the work of Brazilian educator, Paulo Freire (1973), participatory approaches are also underpinned by the notion of 'empowerment'. The Ottawa Charter for Health Promotion (WHO 1986) sees empowerment as a process that enables people to gain more control over the determinants of their health. Freire proposes that empowerment can be achieved through 'critical education', a group dialogue approach that involves a cyclical process of 'discussion-reflection-action' and learning from action. People engage in *discussion* about an issue of concern (sharing and listening to a variety of alternative perspectives and mutually learning from each other), *critical reflection* (thinking about the factors influencing their lives and health, and jointly building a new critical understanding about the underlying social and political causes of their circumstances) and *action* (collaboratively developing strategies to empower themselves to take action). This approach has the potential to transform power relations between individuals, communities, organisations and governments (Minkler & Wallerstein 2010).

Over the last decade, an increasing interest in participatory, community-based approaches to health communication has been occurring in parallel with rapidly changing media environments and communication technologies. To date, much public health media scholarship has been critical of the ways in which health issues and minority/marginalised groups are represented in mainstream media. Many of these studies have argued that limited and stigmatising portrayals of people and their practices contribute to invisibility, discrimination, victim-blaming, resulting in the needs of these communities being systematically ignored (Bowles 2010). There is also a strong and growing literature from media and cultural studies suggesting that mainstream media portrayals of 'vulnerable' groups, such as people living with disability or mental illness, often underestimate their agency, voices and power to draw attention to the challenges of their lives and agitate for change (Holland et al. 2008).

As we have discussed in earlier chapters, contemporary media and cultural studies models emphasise that media audiences are not passive receivers of media content, but are active participants in media consumption and production. The mediation of culture and community is a process of exchange in which meanings are constantly being produced, contested and reproduced by audiences. Audiences are actively engaged in meaning-making and also their own processes of 'media-making'. People themselves become agents of change through their engagement with, and influence on, various media and new modes of communication (see chapters 1 and 2).

Far from being silenced or rendered invisible, a diverse range of minority groups across the world are using digital technologies, the Internet, community media, narrowcasting and social media strategies to share their perspectives, build community and ensure that their voices are heard (see Ellis 2008). Using low-cost, simple digital tools, individuals and communities are creating a diversity of images, video, audio, graphics and text that are easily uploaded, shared and networked. Marginalised groups are also becoming more actively engaged in 'talking back' to mainstream media, challenging mainstream representations and speaking up about issues in their communities (Anderson 2012a; Holland et al. 2009). Importantly, these contributions have the potential to expand the ways diversity and community are experienced and discussed, both in people's everyday lives and in more public debates (Dreher 2010).

Consequently, participatory health communication emphasises the importance of facilitating opportunities for people to become engaged in 'media-making' as a means of representing their perspectives and participating in community change. Most approaches involve building upon the ways in which this is already taking place, through a highly diverse array of community media and online communities (see Chapter 7) and will be the focus of this chapter and those to follow.

First, we will explore some important practical considerations for PHC by examining several case studies that illustrate the use of *Photovoice*, an approach to community-based, documentary photography. Over the last two decades, Photovoice has been used as a tool for building community and communicating about health in a wide range of marginalised communities around the world (Chonody et al. 2013).

How participatory approaches work in practice

Photovoice: Participatory photography for social change

In 1995, health promotion workers Caroline Wang and Anne Burris developed Photovoice as a participatory action research tool while they were working on a women's reproductive and development programme in rural villages of Yunnan, China. They explored the use of community-based photography as a way of engaging and empowering marginalised women in a process of recording and analysing the social conditions of their lives. Photovoice is informed by principles of health promotion, feminist theory and Freire's approach to critical education. The process aims to (1) enable people to record and reflect on their community's strengths and concerns, (2) promote critical dialogue and knowledge about important community issues through group discussion of photographs, and (3) reach community leaders and policy-makers (Wang 2006).

According to Wang (2006), Photovoice is a method that enables people to define for themselves and others, including policy-makers, what is worth remembering and what needs to be changed. Photovoice projects seek to strengthen and empower communities through participation. Around the world, Photovoice has been used to 'give voice' to a wide variety of marginalised and disenfranchised people, helping to build the capacity of their communities to promote change.

For example, in South Carolina, the United States, people living with spinal cord injuries have successfully used Photovoice to advocate for changes to community environments that improve access for people in wheelchairs. By photographing aspects of local environments that are barriers and facilitators to community participation and matching them with stories about how this affects everyday life for citizens with disabilities, they have created a visual evidence-base for policy-makers whilst also ensuring that their voices are heard by decision-makers (Newman 2010). Photovoice is also being used to build community and improve mental health amongst traumatised children living in refugee camps. For example, in Thailand, the *Photofriend* project brings together youth mentors and very young Burmese child refugees separated from their parents. According to Oh (2011), the Photovoice process is helping children to recover from trauma and rebuild a sense of hope, pleasure and play.

Based in Bali, Indonesia, *Photovoices International* is engaging traditional communities in some of the most remote regions of the world in preserving traditional knowledge and documenting the state of natural environments. Photovoice enables community people, many of whom are illiterate and speak only their local language, to directly communicate indigenous knowledge and concerns from the grassroots to international organisations, government officials and the resource industries. By using simple cameras, photographs and stories, the realities of people's lives and their hopes for the future can be represented at the decision-making table (see *www.photovoicesinternational.org*).

How does Photovoice work? Youth violence prevention

This section offers a practical case study to illustrate the use of Photovoice for community-building among youth, adults and policy-makers to address youth violence. It is based on the work of Wang and colleagues (2006, 2004) and leads into more recent multimedia initiatives in the United States and the United Kingdom.

Youth violence in the United States

In 2001, the US Center for Disease Control (CDC) identified youth violence as a critical public health issue (CDC 2010). In 2007, an average of 16 young people between 10 and 24 years of age were murdered each day in the United States, making homicide their second leading cause of death (CDC 2010). Homicide rates for this age group were consistently higher than that for all other age groups combined. According to Chonody et al. (2013), for every person who gets shot and dies, another four are shot and survive. For each person who dies from stab wounds, 64 survive. Behind these horrific numbers are individuals, families and communities, each with their own story. Many are young people of colour living in poverty-affected neighbourhoods. Homicide rates for these young people are 20 times the rate for Whites and nearly three times the rate for Hispanics.

Flint Photovoice: Talking through pictures
Flint and Genessee county is a low-income county of Michigan. Since the collapse of the local automobile industry in the early 1990s, the community had struggled with the process of redefining its economy, culture and race relations, and there was growing concern about violence within the community (Wang et al. 2004). The Flint Photovoice project was initiated by the Neighborhood Violence Prevention Collaborative, a coalition of 265 neighbourhood groups and block clubs. Flint Photovoice involved the work of 41 youths and adults who used Photovoice to photograph community assets and concerns, critically discuss the resulting images and communicate with policy-makers. Using Wang's (2006) Photovoice method as a framework, we briefly describe how the project worked, what it achieved and what factors contributed to its success. We start by outlining the key practical steps involved.

1. *Engaging with policy-makers and community leaders:*
In the early stages, project leaders secured the interest of local policy-makers and community leaders who were likely to be sympathetic to the project and a 'guidance committee' was formed. A small group of policy-makers also agreed to participate as photographers. Although several reported feeling totally out of their depth, they became invaluable ambassadors for the project.

2. *Recruiting participants and planning the project with the community:*
Photographers included youth community leaders, adult activists and policy-makers. Local facilitators and professional photographers were recruited to assist with workshops. Participants were involved in project planning and fine-tuning.

3. *Workshops and skill building:*
Following Photovoice training, facilitators conducted small-group workshops with participants. Early workshops introduced Photovoice methods; the ethics and responsibility that come with using a camera; minimising potential risk to subjects and yourself; and the ethic of giving back photos and expressing thanks. In later workshops, participants brainstormed ideas about initial themes they might use for taking pictures. Cameras were distributed and participants built confidence and skills in basic photography. In Flint Photovoice, disposable cameras were used, but more recent projects lend low-cost digital cameras to participants (Chonody et al. 2013).

4. *Obtaining informed consent:*
Written informed consent forms were completed by (1) participants, (2) people who were photographed and (3) participants consenting to have their photos made public.

5. *Getting out and taking photos:*
Participants agreed on time needed to take pictures, usually one week for each photo shoot. Participants explored their local community, taking pictures of:

o   their everyday health, family and work realities;
o   things in their lives that they want to talk about or change; or
o   to simply show others how they see their world.

6. *Selecting photos, discussion, reflection:*
In small group workshops, participants engaged in a three-step process:

1.   Selecting and talking about photos. Each participant selected two or more pictures that they were comfortable sharing and talking about.
2.   Telling the story of their own photograph by first doing a 'freewrite' (writing captions or a brief narrative) and then explaining to the group what is happening in the picture and what it means to them. The group would then reflect more critically on the picture, with discussions guided by the mnemonic, SHOWeD:

S What do you *see* here?
H What is really *happening*?
O How does this relate to *our* lives?
W *Why* does this problem or strength exist?
D What can we *do* about it?

3.   Identifying and selecting key themes. This photo-taking and critical reflection process was repeated several times over a six-week period, during which participants gradually built a consensus about the most important key themes and how they could be communicated through the pictures and stories.

Participants captured incredible images focused on disused buildings, decrepit public facilities and vandalism, as well as people's experiences of alcohol, drugs, racism, religion, poverty and lack of youth opportunities. Other pictures focused on the hope and resourcefulness of local people and the possibilities found in places such as a community garden, a well-cared for park or a stunning graffiti wall. One participant had photographed her husband standing on a bridge taking a picture of her. Titled 'Looking back at you while you are looking back at me', it suggests how people wanted to redefine how the community saw itself and move beyond its violent reputation. Another, entitled 'Exploded Frustration' taken by 17-year-old Eric Dutro, featured a bullet hole on his bus. Eric wrote:

> Violence. The line of the snow and concrete dividing the bullet hole shows that there are two sides to every story – a person with a gun and demands and a person with fear and a wallet. I am going to school. I can tell that the bus I ride in is always different because the bullet holes are always in different windows... Many people use public transportation... the bullet holes are cold reminders that you never know what will happen next. This

violence exists because people don't know how to deal with hardships and anger. They think it's easier to rob people for money or shoot when they are scared...We need to give people positive confidence somehow. Show them that they have special skills and help them find out what their gifts are. Once they believe that they are not victims of circumstance and they can determine their destiny, they will find this strength many times more powerful than a gun.

(Wang 2006: 913)

7. *Exhibition: Plan with participants a format to share photographs and stories.*
This stage is pivotal for celebrating achievements, building community understandings and generating action. Using their photos and stories, Flint Photovoice participants presented their concerns to policy-makers, community leaders, the media and general public through a local exhibition, a series of invited forums, legislative breakfasts, a display in the city hall and in local and national health departments and news programmes. While Flint Photovoice participants used mounted photographs and PowerPoint shows, more recent youth violence initiatives have also created websites, shared exhibits on Facebook and Flickr and created compelling YouTube 'photovoice' videos. Many of these exhibits have attracted several thousands of views (see also the UK-based www.photovoice.org)

8. *Follow-up and evaluation:*
Developing a plan for action to be taken after the exhibition enables participants to give direction to the next phases of generating change. It is also important to follow-up with individual participants to further build skills, contacts and opportunities to continue their involvement. In Flint, several participants attended follow-up meetings, volunteered for community advisory committees and led local initiatives to address local issues. Participants were involved in evaluating the project's processes and outcomes. Sharing the key lessons learned has made an important contribution to building the evidence-base for participatory projects more generally (Catalani & Minkler 2010).

What were the outcomes and success factors?
According to Wang et al. (2006, 2004), Flint Photovoice enabled youths to express their concerns about neighbourhood violence to policy-makers and to exhibit their work in a range of media and highly visible public forums. Amongst the policy-makers who took photographs, many gained experience with a methodology which they then adapted for other community health programmes. The success of Flint Photovoice was instrumental in gaining funding for a range of longer term initiatives, including a CDC-supported Youth Violence Prevention Centre.

Community-building was facilitated through the participation of people differing widely in age, income, experience, neighbourhood and social power. Through the Photovoice process, which extended over many months, long-term relationships were formed. People no longer saw one another as inaccessible and lacking common ground but instead found new ways to draw on each others' expertise. Flint Photovice also made a substantial contribution to building community capacity for addressing broader issues that influence public health, including quality of neighbourhood environments, economic development, faith-based health initiatives, racism and youth opportunities.

Extending Photovoice for youth violence prevention
In the years since Flint Photovoice, hundreds of Photovoice projects have been used to address youth violence and related issues in the United States, the United Kingdom, Australia, Israel-Palestine, Bosnia, Africa and elsewhere around the world (see Chonody et al. 2013; Wang 2006). Some have extended Photovoice to include community video-making using low-cost digital video-cams, mobile phones and basic digital editing technologies. In London, for example, Photovoice UK has initiated *Look Out!* Initially, in 2010, the pro-gramme worked with young people in supported housing to facilitate their participation in debates seeking solutions to the problem of gangs and knife crime in the inner city. By 2013, the project had been extended to Manchester, Liverpool, Nottingham and Glasgow, creating opportunities for young people to speak out on issues they feel strongly about. Youth-generated photogra-phy, video, music and spoken word performances have been showcased via youth media websites and magazines, viral Internet campaigns and national press. *Look Out!* has created new opportunities for youth to have a legitimate voice at the table, engaging in dialogue and generating solutions along with politicians, policy-makers and community leaders (see www.photovoice.org).

Box 6.1 provides a summary of the practical steps involved in Photovoice. More detail is available in Wang (2006) and Rabinowitz and Holt (2012).

Box 6.1   Photovoice practical steps

1. **Engage** policy-makers and community leaders.
2. **Recruit** participants and plan the project with the community you are work-ing with.
3. **Photovoice workshops** introducing participants to the methods, responsibil-ities and ethics; brainstorming ideas about what might be photographed; basic photography skills to build skills and confidence.
4. **Obtain informed consent** at all three levels: photographers, subjects and permission to publish.
5. **Get out and take photos** to capture the strengths and concerns of this community.
6. **Select/discuss/reflect** workshops; discuss photographs; critically reflect, identify themes.
7. **Exhibition** Share photographs and stories to: celebrate achievements; communicate key themes to wider community and decision-makers; and generate action.
8. **Follow-up and evaluate** to facilitate further opportunities for participants and maintain momentum for using the project to bring about change.

Ethical issues and challenges

Participatory health communication projects take place within contexts where multiple inequalities exist, so it is crucial to ensure that the processes and strategies do not have negative impacts.

Responsible and ethical practice is essential, and the best interests of project participants must always be upheld. In particular, working with children can provide specific ethical challenges. As Lal et al. (2012) note, the moral and privacy rights of young and/or vulnerable people and the use of their images on the Internet – as photographers and as subjects – need to be carefully managed. Photovoice (2009) provides a useful guide for using Photovoice with children. Based on their experience in refugee camps, using Photovoice with child refugees from Burma and Palestine, Oh (2011) and Nakkash et al. (2012) provide valuable practical insights and strategies to protect vulnerable children from further harm associated with opening up traumatic experiences of violence, fear, flight, hunger and pain.

Public exposure through participatory methods, such as Photovoice, can also bring risks as well as rewards. For example, Lal et al. (2012) have reviewed the growing use of Photovoice with people experiencing physical, intellectual and mental disabilities. She reports on several studies in which the authors question whether the Photovoice process, in singling out a particular community, reinforces existing stigmatisation rather than contributing to its reduction. It is important to support participants throughout the process of engaging with various audiences, including the media, so they feel well-prepared and in a better position to maintain control over how the project and participants are represented.

Important practical considerations

Many of the insights from the case study of Photovoice can be applied in other approaches to participatory health communication. With this more general context in mind, the last part of this chapter will draw together important practical considerations and key lessons from practice that are useful for all approaches to participatory, community-based health communication.

As our case studies have shown, participatory approaches are guided by three key practical considerations (Minkler & Hancock 2010):

- Starting 'where the people are'
- Helping communities to identify and build on community strengths and assets
- Using the power of dialogue.

Starting 'where the people are' is the most important element of working with communities. Rather than entering as an outside expert armed with epidemiological evidence and a predetermined idea of what is 'wrong' with a community, it involves listening to what people say about issues of concern in their communities. Starting 'where the people are' demonstrates to the community that their perspectives are respected. It also ensures that the focus is on issues which the community identifies, and feels strongly enough about, that it is willing to work on it to bring about change (Minkler & Hancock 2010). In order to start where the people are, we need to spend time getting to know more about communities, building trust, and developing a deeper understanding of how they see our role as facilitators in their communication processes. This is the pivotal first step towards ensuring that the project will be effective and sustainable.

The second important dimension of participatory practice involves helping communities to identify and build on community strengths and assets. Well-meaning professionals often cause harm to communities by reinforcing a 'deficit mentality' in which the community is viewed in terms of its problems, needs and deficiencies that need to be 'fixed' by outside experts. In contrast, participatory approaches focus on the existing resources within communities that can be mobilised to help them collectively address issues that matter to them. There is now a wide range of tools and approaches that communities may find useful for recognising and building on their existing strengths and assets. These approaches can help to identify community strengths such as informal leaders and natural helpers, existing community groups and partnerships and lessons learned from past experience. They also tap into a wealth of insider knowledge about community dynamics and important aspects of cultural identity, as well as the rituals, celebrations and spaces for contestation and conflict that help to give voice to people's concerns and ideas (Minkler & Hancock 2010).

Lastly, participatory approaches are centred around using the power of dialogue. This involves creating opportunities for people to 'speak up' from their own experiences, share and learn from different perspectives and reflect critically on their situation and its causes. In contrast to traditional 'formative research' often used by professionals to better understand communities, dialogue refers to a continual process in which community members and other stakeholders are engaged in 'co-learning' from each other. Fostering dialogue within communities can help people to discuss their hopes for their communities, decide on issues of greatest concern and identify the most relevant social action for tackling those concerns. Furthermore, this process is often helpful for identifying the people who are motivated to become key players in processes of generating change.

Partnerships, planning and evaluation: Lessons from practice

Partnerships

Partnerships are central to participatory health communication. Building relationships between practitioners and community members, gatekeepers and stakeholders is essential. Participation of these groups in each stage of planning, action and evaluation helps to ensure that all voices are represented, the programme is supported and the potential for opposition is minimised (Stanley & MacLean 2005).

'Stakeholders' can include those people and organisations who may be in a position to influence policy or who work with, and provide services to, people from a specific community. This may include practitioners from welfare services, police and emergency services, health professionals and outreach workers. Other stakeholders may include city council members and other politicians, business people, researchers and journalists. Gathering these people together brings a range of perspectives, experience, skills and resources and it can also have significant resource and cost-sharing advantages. Based on several decades of experience using Photovoice, Wang and Pies (2010) recommend that the interest and participation of policy-makers and key stakeholders should be sought as early as possible in order to provide political will and support for implementing participants' potential policy and programme recommendations. A formalised 'guidance' or advisory committee can also help to achieve this purpose.

'Gatekeepers' are those who have influence over access to community members. They may be community leaders (formal and informal), respected elders, gang leaders, or other people with particular cultural significance such as musicians or sportspeople. Gatekeepers also include those with control over places where people can be reached. This includes places where 'hidden' communities gather together: on the street, in shelters, at community food programmes and other support centres, and also in schools, workplaces, churches, sports facilities and other, less formal recreational spaces. Seeking the support of gatekeepers from the outset can mobilise their role as intermediaries, building trust within the community, generating interest in the project and encouraging community people to become actively involved.

Genuine partnerships provide equitable and fair opportunities for a range of community members to participate. As we noted earlier, communities are rarely cohesive, united groups. They are complex social systems made up of people with diverse interests and often involve unequal power relations. Community workers, faced with time and resource constraints, tend to involve only the most dominant, outspoken, literate and easily accessed members of marginalised communities. The advantage of participatory approaches is that community people are engaged in representing, sharing and discussing their perspectives with others in their communities. Tools such as Photovoice take participants out into streets, homes, worksites and public spaces, taking photos, answering questions about the project and listening to the views of other community members about what should be photographed and why. This provides opportunities to draw on the perspectives of a more diverse range of people, including less visible cultural subgroups and people living on the margins of society, whose voices might otherwise remain unheard.

With this in mind, Israel et al. (2010: 53) suggest several important questions to be explored in the early stages of engaging with communities: Who is the community? How do members define this community for themselves? Who represents the community? Who has influence in this community, and how, and are they involved? Who will be the representatives of this community in any partnership and how will this be agreed upon? Who is defined as being 'outside' the community and not invited to participate? Exploring these questions through community dialogue can help the community to identify any 'missing voices' and decide on strategies to facilitate more fair and equitable participation. For example, Wang and Pies (2010) describe the ways that the limited participation of low-income, single mothers and new parents in community workshops could easily be addressed by holding workshops in the evenings, providing a meal and childcare.

Planning

Planning for participatory approaches involves the general planning steps outlined in Minkler and Wallerstein (2010). The primary difference is the emphasis on involving community members in all stages of the process. This ensures that the community's interests remain central to both planning and evaluation. For example, background research about the health status, behaviours, needs and concerns of communities is traditionally informed by epidemiological data and social science research gathered by 'experts'. Nonetheless, differences often exist between what researchers think is important and what the community identifies as being important.

Participatory approaches complement this formal data and help to broaden the views of 'outsiders' by giving priority to the popular knowledge and insights generated by community people themselves. Participatory processes, such as those we have outlined, have a pivotal role in legitimising the perspectives of community members, gathered and presented in ways that make sense to them. Despite being produced outside formal scientific structures, this knowledge is a vital source of expertise (Wang & Pies 2010).

Considerable time needs to be allowed for the process of building relationships, trust and credibility with communities. Furthermore, practitioners can sometimes find it challenging to accept having less control over strategies and outcomes if their previous experience has been in more traditional, expert-led programmes. Participatory approaches can also be more time-consuming to develop and evaluate because they need to allow time for securing resources and for developing the skills and confidence of community members involved in these processes. According to Israel et al. (2010), this time should be viewed as a key investment. Investing in community partnerships is essential for participatory approaches as it provides the foundation for building the capacity of communities to solve complex problems for themselves, long after any official intervention has ended. For more on the participatory planning process, see Rabinowitz and Berkowitz (2103a).

Evaluation

Evaluation should also be participatory, with community members and other stakeholders playing an active role in planning and conducting the evaluation activities, as well as disseminating the findings. According to Springett and Wallerstein (2010: 200), evaluation always has a political dimension because it is 'intimately tied up with societal priorities, resource allocation and power'. These authors emphasise the importance of considering: Whose values are driving the evaluation? Whose standards are being met by the activities being undertaken and assessed? And, whose needs are being met by the evaluation itself? They also remind us that 'if an evaluation is going to change anything, it has to be perceived as useful by everyone involved, whether a funder, participant or project worker' (Springett & Wallerstein 2010: 200). For this reason, participatory approaches to evaluation attempt to involve all those who have a stake in its outcomes so that the questions asked, and the methods used, yield the kinds of new knowledge that will help them take action to improve practice. Furthermore, including a diverse range of participants in each stage often generates innovative approaches for measuring process, impact and outcomes.

Participatory evaluation is most commonly designed around the action research cycle in which community members and other stakeholders are collaboratively engaged in a cyclical process of 'learning from practice' (Springett & Wallerstein 2010). This involves monitoring processes and outcomes, reflecting on successes and challenges and making adjustments to improve practice. Participants evaluate the effects of these changes and the cycle continues. In participatory evaluation, participants are actively involved in disseminating the findings and celebrating achievements with each other and the wider community, as well as with key stakeholders and decision-makers.

Evaluation results can be used to improve processes used for participatory methods. Wider dissemination of evaluation findings helps to build the evidence-base for the ways participatory projects can be used to bring about change. Rabinowitz and Berkowitz (2013b) offer a list of useful participatory evaluation questions that include the following:

Process:

- What is the most effective recruitment method for participants? For staff and volunteers?
- Did participants gain new skills?
- Was the training adequate and effective?
- Did the work of participants contribute to a better understanding of the issue for the community and/or organisations and decision-makers?

Outcomes:

- Did the project lead to continued action on the chosen issue?
- Did the project lead to changes in conditions in the community?
- In what ways were policy-makers influenced to bring about change?
- To what extent was the project sustained over time?

For more information on participatory evaluation, see Springett and Wallerstein (2010).

Reflecting on the challenges of participatory approaches

For practitioners, participatory approaches often involve ethical paradoxes and dilemmas. We value the community while also wanting to be engaged in changing or improving it. We strive to foreground community voices and input, yet we need to ensure that these are communicated in strategic ways that will facilitate change and achieve outcomes. We need considerable time to build community engagement and dialogue, but we also need to meet timelines for reporting outcomes to agencies and funding bodies. McDermott et al. (2008) suggest that the best way to reconcile these challenges is through balancing short- and long-term needs of all partners, mutual respect and the need (and willingness) to be both supportive and critical.

Israel et al. (2010: 48–52) offer an insightful discussion of these challenges in relation to community-based, participatory research. These authors offer a list of principles that provide an invaluable checklist for anyone interested in developing more participatory approaches to health communication:

1. recognises community as a unit of identity;
2. builds on strengths and resources within the community;
3. facilitates collaborative, equitable involvement of partners in an empowering process that attends to social inequalities;
4. promotes a co-learning and capacity-building;
5. integrates research and action for mutual benefit of all partners;
6. emphasises locally relevant health issues and ecological perspectives;
7. develops participatory systems that involve partners a cyclical and iterative process, responding to feedback and making ongoing adjustments;
8. disseminates findings and knowledge gained to all partners;
9. involves long-term process and a commitment to sustainability by all partners.

CHAPTER SUMMARY

- Participatory approaches are not just about giving people information and telling them things that experts think they need to hear. They are about creating opportunities for engaging in dialogue and working towards shared understandings. They are grounded in listening to people and empowering them to come up with solutions that suit them (Max 2012).

- Participatory approaches actively involve people in: articulating their perspectives, identifying community concerns, selecting issues, critically reflecting on their sources and collaboratively generating solutions and strategies. Important practical considerations include starting where people are at; emphasising and building on community strengths; and using the power of dialogue.

- Participatory, community-based health communication has an important role in helping people take control over the factors that influence their health. This approach helps to build social connection, stronger communities and generate action for social change. Consistent with the WHO Ottawa Charter for Health Promotion (1986), this approach seeks to facilitate opportunities for people to *enable, mediate* and *advocate* for health.

> • In summary, working *with* communities using participatory approaches can strengthen the planning, implementation, evaluation and long-term sustainability of health promotion. When the authority of community members is acknowledged, and they are supported in taking responsibility for communicating about health, new opportunities are also created for their participation in ongoing dialogue with decision-makers, governments, organisations and wider society. Incorporating the cultures, energy and ideas of community people into policy and programme development helps to build a more healthful and democratic society.

References

Anderson, H. 2012a, *Raising the Civil Dead: Prisoners and Community Radio*, Peter Lang, Bern.

Basu, A. and Dutta, M. 2009, 'Sex workers and HIV/AIDS: Analyzing participatory culture-centred health communication strategies', *Human Communication Research*, 35 (1): 86–114.

Basu, A. and Dutta, M. 2011, ' "We are mothers first": Localocentric articulation of sex worker identity as a key in HIV/AIDS communication', *Women and Health*, 51 (2): 106–123.

Bowles, K. 2010, 'Representation', in G. Turner and S. Cunningham (eds), *The Media in Australia*, 3rd Edition, Allen and Unwin, Crows Nest, NSW, 64–77.

Catalani, C. and Minkler, M. 2010, 'Photovoice: A review of the literature in health and public health', *Health Education and Behaviour*, 37 (3): 424–451.

Centers for Disease Control and Prevention. 2010, 'Injury prevention and control: Data and Statistics'. Accessed 6 May 2014 http://www.cdc.gov/injury/wisqars/index.html.

Cheatham-Rojas, A. and Shen, E. 2010, 'CBPR with Cambodian girls in Long Beach, California: A case study', In M. Minkler and N. Wallerstein (eds), *Community-Based Participatory Research for Health: From Process to Outcomes*, Wiley, San Francisco.

Chonody, J., Ferman, B., Amitrani-Welsh, J. and Martin, T. 2013, 'Violence through the eyes of youth: A Photovoice exploration', *Journal of Community Psychology*, 41 (1): 84–101.

Clements-Nolle, K. and Bachrach, A. 2010, 'CBPR with a hidden population: The transgender community health project a decade later'. In M. Minkler and N. Wallerstein (eds), *Community-Based Participatory Research for Health: From Process to Outcomes*, Wiley, San Francisco.

Dreher, T. 2010, 'Cultural diversity and the media', in S. Cunningham and G. Turner (eds), *The Media and Communications in Australia*, Allen & Unwin, Crows Nest, 273–284.

Dutta, M. J. 2008, *Communicating Health: A Culture-Centered Approach*, Polity, London.

Dutta, M. J. 2011, *Communicating Social Change: Structure, Culture, and Agency*, Routledge, New York.

Egger, G., Spark, R. and Donovan, R. 2005, 'Focus on populations: Social marketing and the media', *Health Promotion Strategies and Methods*, McGraw-Hill, Sydney.

Ellis, K. 2008, 'Beyond the Aww Factor: Human interest profiles of paralympians and the media navigation of physical difference and social stigma', *Asia Pacific Media Educator*, 19: 23–35.

Freire, P. 1973, *Education for Critical Consciousness*, Continuum, New York.

Holland, K., Blood, W., Pirkis, J. and Dare, A. 2009, 'Postpsychiatry in the Australian media: The "vulnerable" talk back', *Asia Pacific Media Educator*, June 2008/July 2009, (19): 143–157.

Israel, B., Schulz, A., Parker, E., Becker, A., Allan, A. and Guzman, R. 2010, 'Critical issues in developing and following CBPR principles', in M. Minkler and N. Wallerstein (eds), *Community-Based Participatory Research for Health: From Process to Outcomes*, Wiley, San Francisco, 47–66.

Lal, S., Jarus, T. and Suto, M. J. 2012, 'A scoping review of the Photovoice method: Implications for occupational therapy research', *Canadian Journal of Occupational Therapy*, 79 (3): 181–190.

Lardeau, M., Healey, G. and Ford, J. 2011, 'The use of Photovoice to document and characterize the food security of users of community food programs in Iqaluit, Nunavut', *Rural and Remote Health*, 11: 1680.

Lemelle, A., Reed, W. and Taylor, S. (eds) 2011, *Handbook of African American Health: Social and Behavioural Interventions*, Springer, New York.

Max, J. 2012, 'Student wins Prime Minister's Pacific-Australia Award', *Centre for Communication and Social Change Newsletter*, University of Queensland. Accessed 6 May 2014 http://www.uq.edu.au/ccsc/student-wins-prime-minister-s-pacific-australia-award.

McDermott, V., Oetzel, J. and White, K. 2008, 'Ethical paradoxes in community-based participatory research', in H. Zoller and M. Dutta (eds), *Emerging Perspectives in Health Communication: Meaning, Culture and Power*, Routledge, New York.

Minkler. M. and Hancock, T. 2010, 'Community driven asset identification and issue selection', in M. Minkler and N. Wallerstein (eds), *Community-Based Participatory Research for Health: From Process to Outcomes*, Wiley, San Francisco, 153–167.

Minkler, M. and Wallerstein, N. (eds) 2010, *Community-Based Participatory Research for Health: From Process to Outcomes*, Wiley, San Francisco.

Nakkash, R., Alaouie, H., Haddad, P., El Hajj, T., Salem, H., Mahfoud, Z. and Afifi, R. 2012, Process evaluation of a community-based mental health promotion intervention for refugee children, *Health Education Research*, 27 (4): 595–607.

Newman, S. D. 2010, 'Evidence-based advocacy: Using Photovoice to identify barriers and facilitators to community participation after spinal cord injury', *Rehabilitation Nurse*, 35 (2): 47–59.

Oh, S. 2012, 'Photofriend: creating visual ethnography with refugee children', Area, 44 (3): 382–288.

Photovoice 2009, 'Statement of ethical practice', *Photovoice*. Accessed 6 May 2014 http://www.photovoice.org.

Pullen, C. and Cooper, M. (eds) 2010, *LGBT Identity and Online New Media*, New York, Routledge.

Rabinowitz, P. and Holt, C. 2012, 'Implementing photovoice in your community', *Community Toolbox*, University of Kansas. Accessed 6 May 2014 http://ctb.ku.edu/en/tablecontents/chapter3_section20_main.aspx.

Rabinowitz, P. and Berkowitz, B. 2013a, 'Participatory approaches to planning community interventions', *Community Toolbox,* University of Kansas. Accessed 6 May 2014 http://ctb.ku.edu/en/tablecontents/section_1143.aspx.

Rabinowitz, P. and Berkowitz, B. 2013b, 'Community based participatory action research', *Community Toolbox*, University of Kansas. Accessed 6 May 2014 http://ctb.ku.edu/en/tablecontents/section_1349.aspx.

Springett, J. and Wallerstein, N. 2010, 'Issues in participatory evaluation', in M. Minkler and N. Wallerstein (eds), *Community-Based Participatory Research for Health: From Process to Outcomes*, Wiley, San Francisco, 199–215.

Stanley, D. and MacLean, M. 2005, 'Narrowcast communications', in R. Moodie and A. Hulme (eds), *Hands on Health Promotion*, IP Communications, Melbourne, 84–93.

Taylor, J., Wilkinson, D., Cheers, B. (2008) *Working with Communities in Health and Human Services*. Oxford University Press, Oxford.

Vaughan, C. 2010, ' "When the road is full of potholes, I wonder why they are bringing condoms?" Social spaces for understanding young papua new guineans' health-related knowledge and health-promoting action', *AIDS Care*, 22 (2): 1644–1651.

Wang, C. 2006, 'Youth participation in Photovoice as a strategy for community change', *Journal of Community Practice*, 14 (1): 147–161.

Wang, C., Morrel-Samuels, S., Hutchison, P., Bell, L. and Pestronk, R. 2004, 'Flint Photovoice: Community building among youths, adults and policymakers', *American Journal of Public Health*, 94 (6): 913–911.

Wang, C. and Pies, C. 2010, 'Using Photovoice for participatory assessment and issues selection: Lessons from a family, maternal, and child health department', in M. Minkler and N. Wallerstein (eds), *Community-Based Participatory Research for Health: From Process to Outcomes*, Wiley, San Francisco.

World Health Organization 1986, Ottawa charter for health promotion, in WHO 2009, *Milestones in Health Promotion: Statements from Global Conferences*, WHO/NMH/CHP/09.01, 1–5. Accessed 6 May 2014 http://www.who.int/healthpromotion/Milestones_Health_Promotion_05022010.pdf.

Zoller, H. M. and Dutta, M. J. (eds) 2008, *Emerging Perspectives in Health Communication: Meaning, Culture, and Power*, Routledge, New York.

Community Media and Online Communities: Media-Making

7

Chapter overview

In this book so far, each chapter has emphasised the importance of facilitating opportunities for ordinary people to become engaged in media-making as a means of representing themselves, their communities and cultures. In this chapter, we illustrate the ways this is already taking place through a diverse array of community media and online communities. We explore some of the ways people are creating and using these collective communication spaces and we examine the ways they might be supported, strengthened and sustained.

The chapter begins by examining the roles of narrowcast and community media, using case studies focused on ethnic and indigenous communities. We then take an in-depth look at several community radio projects developed by people with disabilities, and by prisoners, in order to highlight key principles and lessons from practice. The second half of the chapter explores online communities and virtual worlds, providing insights into the diverse ways in which people are creating and maintaining their own spaces for communicating about health. We examine online support groups and patient communities and we explore the innovative ways in which virtual worlds, such as Second Life, are being used by people living with disabilities, chronic illness and post-traumatic stress. We also explore the creative ways LGBTI people are using 'cybersociality' to maintain mental health and well-being and to build a collective political presence aimed at overcoming stigma and discrimination. Throughout the chapter, we discuss contemporary debates, practical challenges and emerging issues.

Introduction to 3C media: Contexts and characteristics

As we noted in Chapter 4, community and citizens' media exist in the fissures between the public media and commercial media sectors. This third media sector, sometimes referred to as '3C media', provides opportunities for citizens to create social dialogue within their communities by telling their own stories and creating their own news and entertainment in ways that are not possible in mainstream media (Salazar 2010).

In contrast to mainstream corporate media, community media are largely not-for-profit, staffed by volunteers and driven by a public interest focus. Community newspapers, radio, television and online communities are often critical and progressive, encouraging activism and attention to social justice issues. In some instances, they enable the structures and institutions of mainstream media to be reoriented and used by local communities to meet their needs and interests. In others, they utilise digital technologies and the online spaces of networked, interactive media to give voice to minority and marginalised groups within their own communities and more globally (Howley 2010).

In recent years, there has been a proliferation of community and citizens' media worldwide as global media industries have become more dominated by corporate interests and profit-making imperatives. Concentration of media ownership has fortified the power of elite individuals and corporations to dominate decision-making about which issues, content and voices are legitimate in mainstream media. Within this context, as media scholar Clemencia Rodriguez (2010) argues, community and citizens' media have an essential role in providing opportunities for less powerful groups of people to access resources for media-making and to use these to strengthen their sense of community, narrate their identities, voice their concerns and express their own visions for a future.

Contexts for 3C media

According to Howley (2010), community media have an important role in a range of settings and contexts. In the United States, they provide a non-commercial alternative to profit-oriented media industries. In Canada, Australia and Western Europe, they offer an alternative to the monopoly of public service broadcasters and their construction of homogeneous national identity. In developing countries, the participatory nature of community media provides opportunities for citizens to take an active role in processes of social change, economic development and building more democratic societies. In countries governed by repressive regimes, they offer alternatives to state-controlled 'official' media. Even in societies with constitutional protection of free speech, such as the United Kingdom, the United States and Australia, 3C media provide important opportunities for local communities create the social spaces and political openings where alternative voices can be expressed and heard.

Defining characteristics of 3C media

3C media have several characteristics that differentiate them from corporate media. These include a focus on access, participation and enacting active citizenship. Access refers to the way the structures and management of 3C media aim to ensure that a wider range of community members have access to media that is relevant and meaningful for their communities. Participation involves creating opportunities for people to build a 'sense of ownership over the means and process of communication' by becoming active participants in the media-making process (Salazar 2010: 57). 3C media offer opportunities for communities and people who are routinely marginalised to move from being passive audiences to active media-makers. In doing so, they discover new possibilities for their voices to be expressed and heard.

Rodriguez (2001) developed the term 'citizens' media' to describe those media that allow people to 'name the world and speak the world in their own terms'. For Rodriguez, citizens' media provide opportunities for people to enact what she calls 'active citizenship' on a day-to-day basis through their participation in everyday social interactions and political practices. In doing so, individuals and collectives can gain access to power, and they can use this power to redirect and shape their communities. The study of 3C media tends to focus less on what people do and say with their media and more on how participation transforms those citizens and their communities. The real strengths of 3C media are to be found in the cultural and social processes that are triggered when communities take greater control over media content and production.

Narrowcast, community and citizen's media

Narrowcast communication provides an alternative to mainstream print and broadcast media. Narrowcast media enable members of a given community (linked by such things as shared values, ethnicity, religion, health experiences, recreational activities, sexuality, political interests, location) to connect with one another, and to share and publish (make public) their news, information, ideas, images and stories. Examples such as ethnic community newspapers, prisoners' radio, online LGBTI communities or remote indigenous community TV all play an important role in building and maintaining community; strengthening people's sense of identity and belonging; and providing a platform for identifying important shared issues, problems and solutions. These communicative spaces are vital for strengthening community cohesion and stability, and also for providing opportunities for change.

While narrowcast and community media can be focused primarily *within* a particular community, they also provide an important springboard for ensuring that the voices and concerns of minority and marginalised groups find their way *beyond* their community of interest and into the broader public sphere. Community and social media create innovative opportunities for the 'missing voices' of marginalised people to become consolidated, mobilised and transferred into mainstream media, providing wider audiences with insights into the everyday realities of their lives. As the range of media perspectives available to mainstream audiences becomes wider and more diverse, new opportunities emerge for exploring the challenges of diversity, breaking down barriers and creating new platforms for social and political change (Dreher 2010).

Community media have provided an important alternative to mainstream commercial and public media for many decades. From their beginnings in small street-press newspapers and niche community magazines to more con-temporary digital radio, TV, the Internet and social media, these media provide communication opportunities for groups who have traditionally been excluded from mainstream media-making processes. Community media are widely recognised as a vital part of a healthy, democratic and participatory public sphere through their role as facilitators of social inclusion and active citi-zenship for people who are poor, socially excluded, stigmatised or otherwise marginalised (Anderson 2012a; Curry Jansen et al. 2011).

Ethnic media: Diaspora communities, migrants and refugees

Ethnic and migrant community media have an extremely important health pro-motion role in maintaining language, culture and connection amongst people in their communities. According to Katz et al. (2012), ethnic and commu-nity media facilitate social inclusion because they enable programmes to cover issues of interest and concern to their specific audiences. Unlike mainstream media that focus on attracting wide audiences, ethnic media can cover issues and news of particularly importance to their specific communities, such as how to enrol young children in schools, or find low-cost or culturally sensi-tive healthcare alternatives. Community media continue to survive, and grow, because they tell the community-focused stories that other media outlets do not (Lin et al. 2010).

Community media are often small and locally produced. Many also use low-cost websites and social media to enhance their interactions with local audiences (Pew Research Center 2012). As a result, community media are able to provide their audiences with locally generated content and pressing issues that larger media networks are either unaware of or do not have the locally based journalists to cover. According to Lin et al. (2010), community media are fundamental to the health of ethnic and refugee communities because they produce culturally relevant, locally focused content that assists residents to connect with community resources, organisations and each other.

Community media can also help translate larger social issues and ideas into local contexts and understandable actions for their audiences (Katz et al. 2012). For example, the Pew Research Center (2009) found that ethnic media played a critical role in the 2008 US presidential election of Barack Obama. These community media encouraged citizenship-eligible immigrants to natu-ralise in time to vote. They also provided information on voter registration and actions new voters could take if they were turned away on Election Day. This example demonstrates the important role community media can play in strengthening civic engagement, community participation and social capital at local levels.

Amongst migrant and refugee communities, community media can also function as a cultural resource, providing opportunities for maintaining lan-guage, heritage and links with 'home'. On the other hand, the interplay between community media and mainstream media provides an important vehi-cle for migrant communities to share their everyday experiences of negotiating cultural differences, developing a new sense of belonging, and building identities that are more hybrid and cosmopolitan (Dreher 2010). As content from community media becomes integrated into the mainstream, the range of media perspectives becomes wider more diverse and new opportunities emerge for building cross-cultural understanding, trust and dialogue – all of which are fundamental to the process of generating shared solutions to health and social inequities.

Indigenous community broadcasting: Remote areas and dispersed communities

Amongst Australia's aboriginal people, indigenous community TV and radio stations are the primary media used in remote and urban areas. According to Meadows and Foxwell (2008), indigenous audiences report that community media create important opportunities for strengthening their sense of cultural identity, belonging and community, particularly as many extended family members are dispersed across thousands of kilometres.

Community broadcasting also plays a powerful transformative role in the lives of aboriginal people. In recent years, these media have made a significant contribution to addressing the alarmingly high rates of suicide and mental illness amongst indigenous Australians through their important community connection role. In Australia, indigenous people comprise 2.5% of the country's population but they represent 40% of the total prison population (AIHW 2011). Isolation for indigenous prisoners can be crippling, and suicide rates for young indigenous men in prison are tragically high. According to Hogg (2002), less than three out of five indigenous prisoners receive visits from their main social contact outside of prison. Many young prisoners say that indigenous community radio provides them with a morale-boosting lifeline: 'Black people talking over the air, people telling the stories of their lives. I like listening to that' (Meadows & Foxwell 2008: 11).

Indigenous participants in research by Meadows and Foxwell (2008) point to the important role of indigenous radio talkback in enabling the stereotyped portrayal of domestic violence in their communities to be challenged and solutions to be discussed more openly. Hearing first-hand accounts and advice from men who have been through the experience is seen by many as an important way of offering solutions:

> A lot of the time kids don't have that positive image of men in our community. That's the other side of it too, giving the young fellas that positive image that they're not all, you know ... into domestic violence. We're doing positive things in the community as well.

(p.11)

Feelings of pride that stem from either hearing and/or seeing indigenous people on local radio and/or television are strongly expressed:

> So every time I listen to 98.9, I hear voices I know from my community – people I know personally and to hear them on a radio station, I think, it's pretty fantastic.

(p.12)

It's really good [to see local indigenous people on TV] and we see other things happening in other [indigenous] communities. People are really happy, too, when they see that. Kids and older people telling stories and kids know what they're doing at other communities.

(p.12)

We've got that grass roots radio happening. Talking to people. Just that grassroots stuff: none of that high, intellectual stuff. Just the Murri way of talking and communicating; that's what I see as really important in that way so that people understand what you're talking about. You're from the same place, the same area, and you know what you're talking about.

(p.17)

In Australia, community indigenous broadcasting relies on the participation of over 4,000 indigenous volunteers (National Indigenous Radio Service 2014). As audiences and media-makers, participation in community broadcasting generates a sense of empowerment that helps to create and sustain community life through a diversity of music, arts, entertainment and community debate. As we will explore in later chapters, the participatory culture of community media makes it both a vital cultural resource and an essential service that has vast potential for health promotion in indigenous communities.

Prisoners' radio and active citizenship: Locked up, but not forgotten

I think it's fair to say I'm institutionalised and sadly with that comes a certain coldness with emotions... And it also carries with it a build up of hate and self centeredness that's just a build-up of frustration. What I've found this program has created in me is a high level of respect and thankfulness for others who take the time out of their lives for my/others benefit, without judgement, and share enough of themselves to make those who participate, and listen, feel like someone...

(Anderson 2012b: 9)

Prisoners are one of the most isolated populations within society. Incarceration denies prisoners their civil rights as well as opportunities for meaningful employment, recreation, pleasure and play. Many prisoners have little contact with the outside world and are rarely visited by family and friends. The incidence of self-harm and suicide amongst prisoners is between 5 and 20 times higher than people living outside prison walls (Prison Radio 2012). In countries with high levels of imprisonment, such as the United States, there are over 7.1 million citizens under correctional control (Prison Radio 2012).

According to Anderson (2012a), the majority of prisoners are only temporarily removed from society, but this segregation erodes their opportunities and confidence to be actively engaged as citizens in the communities where they will be expected to successfully reintegrate. Prisoners' radio can provide crucial opportunities for people 'on the inside' to maintain self-esteem and to stay connected with their families and friends. Engaging with the wider community through community radio provides an important conduit for the process of 'becoming' a good citizen.

While most Prison Radio stations are confined to broadcasting within prisons, in 2012, there were over 37 prisoners' radio programmes around the world, from the United Kingdom, Canada and Australia to Belize, Jamaica, and South Africa, that had taken the radical step of broadcasting from prison to the 'outside world' (Anderson 2012b). *Beyond the Bars* (3CR, Melbourne) and *Souverains Anonymes* (Ontario, Canada) are a few prisoner radio programmes that directly involve prisoners in live broadcasting as the main aspect of their programming. Most others, such as *Locked In* (4ZZZ Brisbane) and *Jailbreak* (Sydney) include pre-recorded voices of those on the inside on a regular basis. A small proportion of programmes allow talkback calls, but rarely in real time. Permission for direct participation of prisoners is generally difficult to negotiate, so many programmes invite prisoner 'letter-writing' as alternative form of participation. According to Anderson (2012b), one listener to *Locked In* wrote to the show every week for the entire ten years of his sentence. After his release, he continued on as a presenter on the radio team.

Most prisoner radio programmes include workshops aimed to help prisoners prepare pre-recorded contributions such as personal stories of prisoners, former prisoners and their families; prisoners' opinions; quiz sessions; music and poetry. Others, such as *Jailbreak,* include innovative health promotion and harm minimisation components (Minc et al. 2007). *Radio Wanno* (London) provides *Inside Education,* a radio production training programme for prisoners that has been so successful that no participants have ever received further custodial sentences following release (Anderson 2012b).

Active citizenship, empowerment and change
As Anderson (2012a) has documented, participation in community radio can help prisoners overcome isolation, provide opportunities to be heard outside the walls of their confinement and empower them to contribute to changing the conditions of their lives. Prisoners' radio contributes to better rehabilitation outcomes and lower rates of recidivism by fostering a sense for prisoners of being 'active citizens' of the outside world. Anderson's research provides compelling evidence that prisoners' radio can be an empowering form of community media practice that recognises prisoners' tenuous position as citizens and engages them in alternative forms of active citizenship.

Furthermore, prisoners' radio fosters prisoners' engagement with the communities in which they will later live and work. Other opportunities for active citizenship are created by providing public service information and involving prisoners in wider community discussions about the conditions of people's lives that heighten social exclusion and provide pathways into crime. Importantly, these broadcasts also create opportunities for the general public to develop a deeper understanding about imprisonment and the penal system, contributing to more informed policy debates about crime, punishment and prevention.

Prison Radio organisations
Over the last decade, prisoners' radio has gathered momentum. Organisations such as the *Prison Radio Association* (UK) have been established to provide

support, guidance and expertise to existing Prison Radio projects and advise prisons interested in setting up radio projects and radio-training facilities (Prison Radio Association 2012) (see www.prisonradioassociation.org). Others, such as Prison Radio (US), aim to bring the voices of prisoner men, women and children into the public domain through their essays, stories, interviews, films and music. Coordinated through a multimedia website, Prison Radio has also produced content for radio stations, film and television for the last 20 years (Prison Radio 2012) (for more information, see www.prisonradio.org).

Media for all abilities: Disability and chronic illness

While many people living with disabilities and chronic illnesses experience restricted mobility and spend long hours confined to home or bed, many have rich and diverse social lives made possible through community media, online social networks and virtual worlds such as Second Life. These media provide powerful opportunities to share strategies for coping and healing, as well as empower people living with disabilities to take active and rewarding roles in community life. Participation in media-making can also create opportunities to celebrate diversity, challenge stigma and discrimination and advocate for political change (Holland 2009) (Plate 7.1).

A diverse array of media is being produced *by* people in disability communities, *for* people living with disabilities and chronic illnesses, their family friends and supporters. Most use low-cost digital technologies to produce live, online digital programming linking local, national and international audiences.

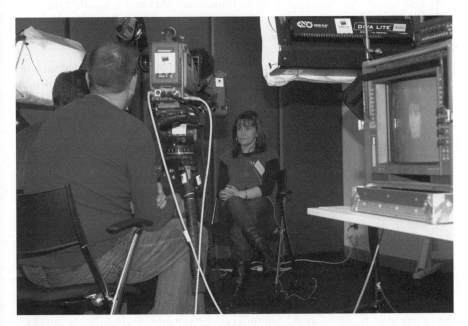

Plate 7.1   Michelle, an ambassador for disability advocacy organisation, Summer Foundation, undertaking media training

Source: Fred Kroh

Digital radio is most widespread because of its low production costs and accessibility for producers, presenters and audiences with limited income and resources. Increasingly, digital video/television and interactive websites are entering this vibrant arena for discussion, debate, humour and play amongst people interested in disability issues. We now turn to two case studies that illustrate the practical steps, challenges and lessons learned in the process of developing community media initiatives for people living with disability.

Able Radio, UK
Able Radio: A Voice for All began in 2006, based in Southeast Wales, and is one of the world's first radio stations run by people living with disabilities. Staffed and managed by a team of volunteers of all ages, most of whom are living with some kind of disability, the station produces live, online, digital radio 24/7, with programmes also available as podcasts to give listeners more accessibility.

Able Radio has grown from modest beginnings. The idea for a small, local radio project originally came from a former radio and television worker whose Type 1 Diabetes and related health, mobility and sensory issues prevented him from continuing to work. Together with a handful of friends who were also passionate about improving the everyday lives of disabled people, the group secured the use of a partly derelict, portable cabin owned by SCOPE services for disabled people in Cwmbran, Wales. With very little money but a mountain of inspiration, they picked up tools, renovated the building and gathered some basic equipment. After deciding on *Able Radio* as their project identity, they established a committee, sought local donations, obtained a small grant from a local trust and began providing training for a group of volunteers who were already using SCOPE services. In no time, a small range of programmes was going to air.

After several months, SCOPE expressed concerns about the difficulty of controlling the quality and content of programmes, forcing Able Radio to seek new sponsorship. So committee members started attending meetings of local networks, councils and charitable funds and eventually found an Entrepreneurs' Fund willing to help them renovate a local day care centre into a wheelchair-accessible studio. As news of the project spread, further community support helped to provide computers, a mixer, microphones and other essential equipment. This also helped Able Radio to make the transition to low-cost digital broadcasting, enabling them to reach larger audiences across the United Kingdom. Careful monitoring, evaluation and reporting of their achievements (as well as lessons learned) have enabled Able Radio to secure the ongoing support of disability organisations, commercial sponsors, charities and local governments around the country (Symons 2010).

The sustainability of the station depends on commitments from volunteers in roles as presenters, producers, researchers, technicians and coordinators. High-quality training workshops with media professionals are provided on a regular basis to build volunteers' confidence and skills in production and presentation. For many participants, this has been a life-changing experience:

Being involved in this fabulous project has given me direction and purpose, a reason to get up each morning and a huge desire to bring hope to so many others who, like me, were lost, feeling useless and overwhelmed by their illness and disability.

Sally M, Able Radio's longest serving presenter (Symons 2010: 6)

I heard of Able Radio when they came to our team meeting, and wondered if it might be of interest to Eiyrion. The young man in question has Aspergers syndrome and has become obsessed with computer games, and has hardly left the house for years. He was persuaded to come to the studio to review games for a programme. In the course of the programme he became increasingly animated and broadened to talking about other subjects. By the end of the interview, he expressed a desire to return and take part in producing programmes at Able Radio regularly. I have worked with him for several years, and never seen him so enthusiastic about anything. I am not ashamed to admit that I stood in the studio and cried.

Julie S, Youth Team Worker (Symons 2010: 6)

The workshops have also been developed as training modules which are now rolled out around the country for other communities interested in producing online radio, generating much-needed revenue for the station. Along with a large grant from the Big Lottery, the Able Radio funding model now includes a unique combination of sponsorship, training and commercial activities.

With a potential audience of 7.5 million people in the United Kingdom living with disability or chronic illness and another six million carers, the station has established itself as the heart of the disability community. Able Radio was producing a range of music, news and current affairs and talk shows with an emphasis on ability-in-disability and a healthy dose of good humour. Other special interest programmes include 'Airing Pain', providing information and support for people living with chronic pain and 'Carers World' offering insights into the world of carers with topical debate and news for carers, family members and friends (Able Radio 2012).

Able Radio also provides a conduit for small disability groups experimenting with producing their own digital content on home computers. In 2012, an Able Radio volunteer read a post on the media blog, *Media UK.com*. It was from the coordinator of a small radio show called 'Shut UP and Listen!' broadcast in Brighton by a group of musicians and DJs with learning disabilities. The group had secured funding from a local charity to produce content for up to two years and were seeking ways to expand their audiences. While commercial stations had shown no interest in taking them on, Able Radio enthusiastically embraced this new partnership and the programme is now 'on air' with a regular timeslot. For more information, go to http://www.ableradio.com/

Ramp Up!
An alternative model has been adopted in Australia with *Ramp Up!*, an online community initiated in 2012 by Stella Young, a community television show host, comedian and professionally trained journalist from the disability

community, in partnership with the ABC, Australia's independent national broadcaster. The *Ramp Up!* website is an 'online meeting place' between mainstream and disability-specific media coverage. The site provides links to all disability-related stories and shows broadcast on ABC TV stations, radio programmes and websites across the country and overseas.

Ramp Up! is a destination for news, discussion, debate and humour, and a lively online community where everyone in Australia's disability communities, family, friends, workers and supporters can have their say. The site also features regular columnists and contributions from people with disabilities, active forums, dynamic video content and many other interactive features to make participation easier. Users of the site are welcomed to create and add their own content and post ideas for improving the site's accessibility, such as close-captioned video for people with hearing impairment. Audiences are asked to encourage other users to join the community and invigorate public ramp up discussion about disability in Australia (ABC 2012).

Ramp Up! is committed to fostering public understanding that communities of people living with disabilities include a diverse range of people. Within these communities, there are lively debates over language, culture and identity: some people are happy to refer to themselves as being 'disabled', while others define themselves as 'living with a disability'. Some people prefer not to identify as having a disability at all. Many community members want a focus on their 'ability in disability', playing down the aspects of their bodies that are different to the mainstream. Others call for greater visibility of their differences and a stronger, more radical, focus on the reality of their conditions and the struggles of their everyday lives (Ellis 2008). Rejecting political correctness and the idea of 'one community voice', the essence of *Ramp Up!* is in creating the space for social interaction and conversations that build respect for the complexity and variety of people in disability communities (ABC 2012). For more information, go to www.abc.net.au/rampup.

Online communities and virtual worlds

Interactive, digital media in health promotion

Digital technologies, the Internet and social media create valuable opportunities for collaborating with communities to identify needs, develop communication strategies and disseminate these within their communities. Social media and Web 2.0 are terms that are often used interchangeably to refer to the loose collection of technologies and services that allow end-users to interact within online communities, share information and collaborate as content creators (Gold et al. 2012). Social networking sites (SNS) offer a novel environment for health promotion due to their popularity, interactivity and potential to engage and create communities.

As we noted in chapters 2 and 3, people are no longer the 'passive' audiences imagined by earlier approaches to health communication. Nonetheless, according to Gold and her colleagues (2012), many public health organisations are finding it challenging to move beyond the one-way information flow of traditional websites to embrace the interactivity and other new functionalities provided by Web 2.0.

Public health organisations and health promotion agencies are increasingly integrating Facebook, Twitter, LinkedIn, MySpace, YouTube, smartphone apps and a range of blogs into their health communication strategies. However, most use more traditional, top-down approaches in order to maintain their control of the way sites are used by audiences. Information tends to be delivered 'out' to audiences, or 'end-users', with opportunities for them to comment and share (Gold et al. 2012). A further degree of control over site activity is maintained by using peer moderators and/or professional staff associated with the programme or intervention (CDC 2012a, 2011).

While giving an impression of being an online community (for example, the US CDC has up to 50,000 'friends' on its social media sites), most public health organisations use social media primarily as an effective, quick and inexpensive method for such things as:

- disseminating information to wide audiences;
- targeting persuasive behaviour-change messages to specific groups;
- marketing and improving relationships with audiences and the public (Parvanta 2011).

However, there is only limited published research describing interventions that use social media in ways that are genuinely interactive and collaborative, involving end-users as co-creators of content. A team of youth and sexual health researchers in Australia have presented an excellent overview of some of the challenges and lessons learned from their research around developing and evaluating interventions using SNS (Gold et al. 2012). The authors also provide a set of detailed recommendations about how to manage some of the tricky practical, technical, ethical, legal and organisational issues that inevitably arise when social media interventions involve sharing user-generated content. Alisa Pedrana and colleagues (2013) provide an in-depth profile of one of their projects exploring the use of SNS to deliver sexual health promotion to men in gay communities. *Queer as F**K* is a video soap/comedy series focused on sexuality, relationships and mental health developed by the Melbourne gay community, in partnership with several award-winning actors, a creative production company and a community organisation. 'Webisodes' were delivered using YouTube and Facebook, and viewers were encouraged to engage, interact and generate content through posts, polls and questions.

While SNS are most often being utilised by public health organisations in a top-down manner, social media are opening up spaces for more grassroots action and interactive health promotion projects. We illustrate this potential below by exploring a selection of these online communities.

Online support groups

Beyond the professional sphere, a variety of blogs and other social media sites are being used by individuals to create and maintain their own support groups and online communities. The Internet is home to a diverse array of small, blog communities, focused on specific conditions and experiences. For example, the blog *Four Walls, No Limits* began in 2010 with 25 followers using the tag 'Surviving and thriving for people who are bedbound, housebound, or anyone else stuck in one place'. The blog discusses pain management, medication, useful products for coping with life in bed, staying entertained and managing stress and loneliness. Blogs like these tend to be small, mutually supportive patient communities with no institutional or commercial affiliations. Nonetheless, *Four Walls* has now expanded into a larger community, with over 2,000 hits per month (URLPulse 2012). The site is linked to a range of related online community groups and carries small-scale, targeted advertising for products such as mindfulness meditation CDs and tapes; books and guides to living with chronic illness; and specialty retailers such as 'No Pity City: Disability gear with slogans that tell it like it is' (see nopitycity.com).

Some critics express concern that SNS are providing new opportunities for commercialisation and exploitation of the spaces where vulnerable people are expressing their health concerns. However, the rapid expansion of community support groups on SNS suggests that these debates are by no means resolved. In Australia, for example, Pedrana et al. (2013) report that SNS and online communities were instrumental in the extraordinary popularity of *Queer as F**K*, the online soap series used to promote conversations amongst gay men about sexual health. Viewers from over 50 countries accessed the videos through online SNS. By series 3, Saudi Arabia had taken over the United Kingdom as the third country with the most video views, suggesting that even in countries where homosexuality attracts the death penalty, these online communities provided supportive cultural spaces where men can interact without feeling intimidated by the possibility of exploitation or surveillance by authorities.

Online patient communities

Large online patient communities, such as *PatientsLikeMe* and *CureTogether*, describe themselves as using 'crowd-sourcing' to provide a space for people with similar health conditions to share stories of coping and recovery, evaluate various healthcare options and exchange useful information. With over 220,000 members in 2013, *PatientsLikeMe* also includes a data-sharing platform which allows members to record data about their conditions, treatment history, side effects, hospitalisations, symptoms and more on an ongoing basis. The site has links with universities and research institutions who use the data to generate new knowledge and to recruit patients for controlled trials (Patients Like Me 2013).

Along with their considerable popularity, sites like these have also been criticised for their 'for-profit' business model and the potential influence of their links with major pharmaceutical companies and other commercial interests. Cancer specialist David Gorski (2012) discusses the promises and pitfalls of profit-oriented organisations such as *PatientsLikeMe*. He argues that despite its admirable core values, such as putting patients first, promoting transparency and fostering openness, this patient 'community' is also a company that is effectively selling a 'product' to partners and investors. The product is a platform containing analyses of testimonials, purportedly from thousands of patients, about their experiences with various medicines and treatments. Gorski argues that the information on the site is not only unsystematic and unreliable but it is also potentially dangerous:

> In essence, PatientsLikeMe is a social media company for patients, that mines the reported experience of its patients as, if you believe the hype, thousands of 'N=1' clinical trials.

(p.1)

In his view, this platform is not only an extremely valuable marketing tool for the businesses who purchase it, but it also has the potential to encourage, directly or indirectly, people making health decisions based on data that is highly preliminary.

Selling sickness through online patient communities

Online patient communities provide numerous industries with access to many thousands of people, creating ever-expanding opportunities to influence the medicalisation of ordinary conditions and everyday life. As we noted in Chapter 4, critical commentators such as Ray Moynihan and Alan Cassels (2005) have provided illuminating research to expose the strategies used by some of the world's biggest drug companies to systematically contribute to the medicalisation of ordinary conditions, widen the boundaries that define illness and increase the markets for medication. Mild problems become redefined as serious illness and common complaints are labelled as medical conditions requiring drug treatments. By widening the boundaries of illness and lowering the threshold for treatments, the pharmaceutical industry is creating millions of new patients and billions in new profits, in turn threatening to bankrupt healthcare systems in many countries.

Numerous industries benefit from expanded markets for tests and treatments (including drugs) and pharmaceutical industries have wide-reaching influence within the medical and healthcare professions. Driven by their vested interest in overdiagnosis, these companies provide funding for direct-to-consumer advertising; establish research foundations to provide evidence supporting their products; sponsor medical education; and conduct strategically targeted 'disease awareness' campaigns through news and current affairs. These industries also exert their influence by sponsoring a wide range of online forums, support groups and patient communities, often using 'astroturfing' in which employees create false online identities and feed into online discussions in ways that promote their corporate interests. Not surprisingly, many of these sponsored groups tend to be quick to celebrate new treatments and technologies but much slower to publicly criticise their limited effectiveness, excessive cost or less publicised side effects (Moynihan et al. 2012).

Online activist communities

In the *British Medical Journal*, Moynihan (2011) argues that a key factor in making health systems more accountable is an educated and informed citizenry – groups of people who are willing to take an active role in debates and community action to influence healthcare and public health decision-making.

Online communities and patient groups provide people with important opportunities to share their concerns, raise awareness of key issues and work collectively together to challenge the power of vested interests in medicine and health care. For example, a number of online citizens' groups have recently emerged with a focus on exposing misleading information and marketing by corporate interests. Some have targeted doctor's associations, while others have set their sights on decision-makers in the pharmaceutical and private health insurance industries (Moynihan et al. 2012). Groups such as *Healthy Skepticism* have helped to expose misleading corporate marketing in the media.

The work of these organisations has also inspired online activist groups from within the medical and healthcare professions. One example, *PharmaPhacts*, is an online community that originated from a small group of politically minded medical students who were concerned about the unhealthy influence of the pharmaceutical industry on medical education. *PharmaPhacts* supporters raise awareness and share information about strategies for student activism, such as taking direct action at university to boycott the equipment, seminars and events sponsored by the pharmaceutical industry. Through their social media networks, their online communication strategies have also attracted media coverage exposing the incentives and lavish gifts to prescribing doctors. One article, titled, 'Spoonfuls of sponsorship making medical students sick', also focused public attention on the broad range of other corporate tactics used to influence healthcare policy and funding (Miller 2009). From humble beginnings, online activist communities like *Healthy Skepticism* and *PharmaPhacts* have mobilised like-minded citizens around the world. Internationally, there is now an established network of online coalitions committed to exposing and challenging unhealthy corporate practices. To learn more, visit http://healthyskepticism.org and Corporate Accountability International http://www.stopcorporateabuse.org.

These online communities are a potent force for change and they are increasingly being recognised as valuable contributors to policy-making and decisions about health care and public health (Laverack 2013).

Virtual worlds: Exploring the possibility of a second life

Virtual worlds can complement the lives of people who are isolated, enriching their quality of life by providing them with outlets for personal creativity, making virtual products, doing jobs that offer real-world payment or by simply giving them opportunities to connect with other people (Best & Butler 2012). For people living with disabilities, virtual worlds provide opportunities to socialise without emphasis on physical appearance, the gaze of others or the stigma they often experience in their 'real' lives (Forman et al. 2011). Virtual worlds are now being used by many people as alternative ways to access information, find social support, enjoy entertainment and explore new experiences without being limited by their disabilities. Consequently, they are also becoming more integrated into rehabilitation and health care (Stewart et al. 2010).

The ME/CFS centre community: Overcoming isolation and loneliness

In an innovative partnership, media researcher Kirsty Best, along with a group of men and women living with chronic health conditions, has created an online community located in the virtual world, called *Second Life*. The *ME/CFS Centre* site is a resource and support centre for people with Myalgic Encephalomyelitis/Chronic Fatigue Syndrome and other invisible illnesses such as Fibromyalgia, Post Traumatic Stress Disorder and Gulf War Syndrome (see Best & Butler 2014).

The ME/CFS Centre mission is to maintain a friendly and calm community within Second Life. It also seeks to raise public awareness about these invisible, and often misunderstood, illnesses. Within this Second Life world, people can explore ways to overcome their social isolation and loneliness. Members of the community create an avatar (or virtual persona) that appeals to their sense of identity and imagination. The avatar can be anything from a tiny cartoon character to a superhero, small child or voluptuous woman, and it becomes their representative as they enter a virtual 3D graphics environment. The avatar can move through the environment, manipulate objects and participate in everyday activities that most people take for granted, such as walking, dancing, conversation and creative activities. Through their avatars, people can interact with others and explore the *Second Life* world, facilitated by text and/or audio.

The ME/CFS Centre in Second Life holds regular meetings, where people gather to find support, friendship and information. They can join real-time chat support groups, listen to visiting speakers and access user-friendly information concerning research and treatment protocols for their condition. Community members can attend guided meditation classes and participate in events such as creating artworks and sharing them in a walk-through virtual exhibition open to the public, family and friends. Links are provided to 'member-contributed resources' as well as their real-life blogs and other social media pages.

People with chronic health conditions often experience spatial and cognitive difficulties, which make it difficult for them to learn how to use and navigate Second Life. This means that stepwise mentoring within Second Life is needed in the early stages to help new users settle in. Most people find that once they overcome these challenges, the benefits of social interaction with people who share their experiences are worth the effort:

I am too sick to function in the real world, but Second Life gives me just that – a chance to interact with people and alleviate the worst effects of severe isolation, in combination with a sense of being in the world . . . albeit virtual [Alex, Male ME/CFS Centre user].

(Cremorne 2010)

Importantly, Centre members are also actively engaged in research to identify accessibility difficulties within Second Life and find new ways to improve the experiences of others (Best & Butler 2012). For those unable to make the journey to Second Life, the Centre website replicates the majority of the information that is provided 'in-world' and a Facebook site provides alternative ways to participate in this creative and supportive online community. To explore the ME/CFS Centre in Second Life, go to http://www.mecfscentre.org.

GimpGirl: Redefining disability

Other related Second Life worlds include *GimpGirl*, a Second Life community for women with various kinds of disabilities (Cole et al. 2011). *GimpGirl* was started in 1998 by Jennifer Cole and several other women with disabilities who 'didn't feel like there was a community out there that understood them and their needs'. According to the *GimpGirl* Mission Statement:

> GimpGirl's mission is to bring women with disabilities together in the spirit of support, positivity and inclusivity. The world of women with disabilities is a complex place, often with no easy answers. We encourage an attitude of self-advocacy and self-efficacy with all of our members and are radically inclusive of all women with disabilities. With the strength of our members and allies throughout the global disability and women's worlds, we use the tools at our disposal to create a place for discourse, humour, art, research, resources, and most of all, community.

(GimpGirl 2014)

The name, *GimpGirl*, aims to stimulate discussion and strip away the sense of stigma and pity surrounding disability: 'Our smart, sassy, sexy members come together to collaborate and share their lives, experiences, problems and successes, in a safe space that focuses more on their commonality as women' (GimpGirl 2014).

GimpGirl welcomes women of all ages, colour, backgrounds and sexual orientations. Through their avatars and the virtual world of Second Life, *GimpGirl* members are actively creating a safe and open space to build community. Through these social interactions, women can experiment with notions of self and identity outside the limitations of mainstream expectations. According to Cole et al. (2011), *GimpGirl* members value the process of 'striving to be of assistance to others', not only because it is inherently satisfying, but also because the role of peer moderator is a means of increasing their own autonomy, freeing them from the role of passive and dependent recipients of services.

To this extent, *GimpGirl* offers opportunities for women to challenge the boundary between 'abled' and 'disabled,' and move beyond stereotypical images of women with disabilities being a docile population with limited needs and aspirations, and who are easily silenced. *GimpGirl* creates a space for these women to redefine the meaning of living with disability and to challenge their double-marginalisation, both as women and as individuals with disabilities (Cole et al. 2011).

Virtual Ability: Rehabilitation and returning to work

Virtual Ability Island is a Second Life world that aims to support people with real-world disabilities, including veterans and people with traumatic brain injury, to build confidence and skills for employment. Originating in Colorado in 2008, the Island provides 'residents' with mentoring, skills training, a virtual Career Fair and demonstrations of assistive technology for the workplace, in order to help to build people's confidence. Other areas on the island, such as 'Match Maker', help to connect job-seeking people living with disabilities to mentors and potential employers in the Second Life world (Stewart et al. 2010). More experienced residents can learn additional skills including photography, creating a profile and managing virtual-world money. The island also contains two small classrooms for training and discussion groups and a large accessible auditorium for community meetings and practising presentations.

The disability support organisation, *Virtual Ability Inc.*, has also adopted the Second Life world *HealthInfo Island*, a consumer health library on topics of physical, emotional and mental health. Librarians who contribute to *HealthInfo Island* are exploring the provision of consumer health information services in a virtual environment through interactive displays, links to outside resources, group events and personalised assistance. For more information, go to http://healthinfoisland.blogspot.com.au/

Virtual worlds, health and happiness

While virtual worlds can help people access information and practical skills, cybersociality also offers unique opportunities for people to experience friendship, kindness, love, family and community. To this extent, virtual worlds have significant consequences in 'real' social life.

In the process of creating a personal avatar, taking on their identity and exploring the world from this new perspective, people are discovering a myriad of possibilities for transcending the limitations of everyday 'real' life and experimenting with notions of self and identity (Cole et al. 2011). They are finding new ways of living with disability and illness; coping with trauma, grief and loneliness; finding pathways to recovery; exploring alternative genders and sexuality; and enjoying relationships in ways they might never have imagined possible. As Boellstorff (2008) notes, 'In virtual worlds we are not quite human – our humanity is thrown off balance, considered anew and reconfigured through transformed possibilities for place-making, subjectivity and community' (p.5).

Research to better understand the possibilities and challenges of virtual worlds for enriching health and happiness is still evolving. But, as this research unfolds, there is no doubt that it will make an important contribution to the future of health communication. For readers interested in a more probing and insightful examination of people's diverse experiences of Second Life, see Tom Boellstorff's (2008) book, *Coming of Age in Second Life: An Anthropologist Explores the Virtually Human.*

Challenges and emerging issues

Recent literature had identified a range of challenges associated with using virtual worlds in health communication (see Best & Butler 2012). This section will discuss three of these: exclusion, impairment and protection. While online technologies are inclusive and widely accessible for many people because they 'reach into where they are', initiatives using virtual worlds also potentially exclude people without basic levels of 'digital literacy' and access to computers and broadband. For people who are both isolated through illness and/or disability and marginalised through poverty and disadvantage, virtual worlds are even less accessible.

Physical impairments create challenges for communication between people using virtual worlds. Depending on their type of disability or health condition, individuals can have very different audio and textual communication needs and abilities. Communication between people with differing visual, hearing and physical limitations is particularly difficult. For example, a person with chronic fatigue syndrome (CFS) may experience difficulty with fine motor coordination needed to type text communication. The introduction of voice communication can enhance his/her ability to communicate, but it poses new difficulties for people with hearing impairment and limits the possibilities for these two people to interact in real time. According to Best and Butler (2012), current modes of live chatting often privilege one sense over the other, and this inability to effectively blend audio and textual communication creates an additional barrier for participants seeking to use technology as a means of communicating with one another. The authors' current research is studying the accessibility requirements of individuals with divergent types of impairment, so that improvements can be made to the accessibility of existing virtual world sites.

The third challenge relates to protection of users. Many Second Life communities have tried to increase accessibility and expand their communities by including more open-source components to their sites, such as Facebook and other social media. However, these complex, mixed-reality environments break down the walls that protect participants from interference by 'outsiders', such as disability fetishists, medical role-players, predatory individuals and commercial interests. They also intensify the need for strong codes of conduct around respect and responsible use by participants. In some cases, moderators have been introduced to help protect the interests and safety of vulnerable community members (Cole et al. 2011).

Nonetheless, attempts to create a safe environment often have the potential to be exclusionary and restrictive. Accordingly, many virtual world communities are also exploring ways to 'reach outside their walls' in order to link with other communities of interest. This also creates opportunities for building new partnerships with service providers and professional groups. By expanding their reach, online communities are building their capacity for working collectively to voice their issues and concerns in the wider public sphere and to advocate for public support and policy change.

Sexual diversity, identity and online communities

Across the world, people of diverse sexualities are participating in a range of online communities within which they gather information and support. Online social networking also provides opportunities for sharing, producing and exchanging ideas, information, music, photos, videos and a vast array of other creative content. For some LGBTI people, online environments and virtual worlds are particularly important because they provide a safe, anonymous space for self-representation, exploration and connection with others with minimal likelihood of unwanted disclosure, disapproval, intimidation or violence (Pullen & Cooper 2010). Furthermore, in comparison to mainstream broadcast media, social media provide a more open arena for LGBTIs to draw attention to inequality and oppression, challenge institutional discourses and reach out to people in need of intimacy, support, information and advocacy (Gillett 2003).

Pullen and Cooper (2010) have published a comprehensive collection of studies exploring the creative ways that people with diverse sexualities are using the Internet and social media to maintain mental well-being, nurture relationships and strengthen their sense of community. The personal stories told by LGBTI people, from a variety of ages, ethnic groups and cultural backgrounds, provide insights into the significance of these online spaces for health and well-being.

The Internet and social media provide opportunities for LGBTIs to explore identity, community and citizenship through:

- connecting to and constructing online communities (at a local and global level);
- exploring opportunities for coming out, such as posting YouTube videos;
- composing self-narratives through blogging and Webcams;
- exploring different aspects of sexual orientation, gender identity and self-representation;
- experimenting with new identities and desires;
- locating explicit sexual health information, including online entertainment-education;
- posting and responding to personal ads to locate romantic or intimate partners;
- courtship conversations, online dating and rehearsal through virtual sex play;
- evaluating preferred employers, health service providers and consumer goods (Pullen & Cooper 2010).

We now turn to two case studies to illustrate the significance of online communities for LGBTI people in a little more detail.

Lesbians married to men

The online environment provides important opportunities for safe self-disclosure within supportive virtual communities. This is particularly the case for lesbians who are married to men. For any woman who is married to a man, and perhaps also has children, finding herself attracted to other women can create a difficult situation. Listening to the experiences of women from around the world, Cooper (2010) provides insights into the ways these women are joining online lesbian communities where they can ask questions, share experiences and gather advice from other women who have been in similar situations.

Many lesbians married to men are living in isolated, rural or religious communities with traditional gender roles and belief systems about marriage and family. Consequently, they have few opportunities to share their questions and concerns about love, loyalty, family and the best interests of their children. For these women, online communities provide a safe space where they can discuss feelings and test identities in a supportive, non-judgmental context. Their coming-out stories suggest these online spaces offer an extremely important sounding board for working out issues before doing so in their families and community, where the consequences may be very high. The support provided through the online community has helped many women to negotiate their lives, and those of their families, in non-traditional ways to create alternative systems for stable, loving relationships. Cooper's research suggests that there are still many unexplored possibilities for online communities in creating mutually supportive spaces for people who feel they don't fit with conventional LGBTI narratives and identities.

Gay and bisexual people in military service

The second example explores online communities as one of the few spaces where gay and bisexual servicemen can express their sexuality without risk of persecution. In 2012, there were over 5,000 lesbian, gay and bisexual people in active military service in diverse locations worldwide (Outserve 2014). Prior to this time, the US military has banned openly gay, lesbian or bisexual persons from military service for many decades. LGBTI people in military service were expected to be silent and compliant with its openly homophobic and discriminatory policies, such as the insidious 'Don't ask, Don't Tell' policy instituted in the 1990s. The stigma, discrimination, bullying and more serious hate crimes during the era of this policy have taken a serious toll on the health and well-being of thousands of young men and women.

Nonetheless, this policy was not able to entirely subdue the energy and creativity of gay servicemen. Tsika's (2010) study documents the ways that same-sex attracted men serving in the US military during this era were able to use the online gay networking site *RealJock.com* to form and maintain community and respond to gay hate crimes. Most were young (between the ages of 18 and 20) and in active service in hotspots, such as Iraq and Afghanistan. His research also shows that the *RealJock.com* community provided an opportunity for gay civilian bloggers and ex-servicemen to support their compatriots serving overseas through conversation, pleasure and virtual sexual play. Blog posts often focused on the aesthetic dimensions of the fitness and muscle-building required to maintain active service – a small compensation for the horrors endured by young servicemen. Importantly, the *RealJock.com* community provided a 'hidden' space for gay servicemen to interact in ways that the Don't Ask, Don't Tell policy could neither limit nor control. This long-standing policy was repealed by President Barack Obama in late 2011 after extensive lobbying by *Outserve*, along with other LGBTI organisations, their families and supporters (Outserve 2014).

Staying negative: Gay men's real stories

Online communities provide an important arena for health communication driven by communities themselves. *Staying Negative* is a campaign supported by the Victorian AIDS Council that taps into the communicative spaces already being used within online LGBTI communities (VictorianAIDS Council 2014). Most HIV-prevention strategies for gay men have traditionally focused on providing men with information that will encourage them to adopt safe-sex behaviours. In reality, safe-sex practices are influenced by a whole range of environmental and cultural factors. *Staying Negative* uses online storytelling to explore these influences on sexual health and broader health issues amongst men who have sex with men (MSM).

Developed *by* gay men *for* gay men, the site has been gathering and sharing stories since 2004. It features over 60 gay and bisexual men telling their own real-life stories about coming out, first sexual experiences, open relationships, and the challenges of negotiating safer sex. The site also provides an opportunity for HIV-positive men to share stories about their lives and how their strategies for staying HIV negative were not successful.

While HIV and safe sex is an important part of these stories, it is not the exclusive focus. The stories do have links to more specific information about reducing HIV/STI risks, relationships and negotiating safer sex (including the four T's), as well as issues surrounding drugs, depression and domestic violence. The site is open to all, it's explicit, there are no restrictions on language or images, and everyone is welcome to submit their story. Links are also provided to support groups, news, events, workshops, peer education opportunities, new research studies and other ways to be involved. To learn more about this innovative approach, go to http://stayingnegative.net.au/.

Staying Negative builds on earlier community-based sexual health communication developed by Victorian AIDS Council that also used storytelling as a central focus. One of these, *Protection,* was initiated for high-risk, gay men who participate in recreational drug use, group sex, sex parties and attending 'sex on premises' venues. Through a more hard-hitting and explicit website, *Protection* shared stories from over 100 men about their own experiences with what they referred to as 'adventurous sex'. The website and print materials also featured professional porn actors who had generously donated their time as models for a variety of explicit images of naked men having sex in different ways. The photos were also tagged with brief, creatively positioned, safe-sex messages. Printed up as pocket-sized booklets and postcards (in which the 'scratchy' safe-sex message could be removed by rubbing with a coin to expose a condom-clad penis), *Protection* resources were distributed by peers in a range of places frequented by other high-risk gay men. Ongoing awareness about *Protection* was also maintained through ads in the gay community media (Victorian AIDS Council 2014).

Sexual diversity, political engagement and social change

While online communities provide important spaces for entertainment, social support and health promotion, they also offer diverse opportunities for LGBTI people to engage politically with wider society, 'presenting themselves to a public as a politically oriented identity'. Pullen and Cooper (2010) argue that, while there is much fragmentation and diversity within LGBTI identities, social media provide opportunities for 'active citizenship' and a collective political presence aimed at overcoming oppression, stigma, discrimination and disconnection:

> ... The new representatives of political power might be the new media producers, engaging in citizenry through the internet, challenging the direct and oppressive power of hetero-normativity.
>
> (p.5)

While this power may be expressed through dissenting LGBTI voices, direct political action and advocacy, it also flows through the diverse expressive and performative spaces of the LGBTI online world that help to create, sustain and celebrate community identities. Within online arenas, a rich tapestry of connections are being made between self and community through visual arts, photography, graffiti, music, live webcams, video and film-making, and simply through time spent talking together. Through their intimate disclosures, personal story-telling, public exhibition, transgressive ideas and stories of change, members of LGBTI communities are creating new opportunities to celebrate diversity and contribute to social transformation.

Understanding this diversity of online LGBTI identities and communities provides important insights into the ways these collective communication spaces might be supported, strengthened and sustained.

Online communities: Emerging issues and challenges

While online spaces create a myriad of opportunities for health promotion, it is important to be mindful of the growing body of literature that challenges utopian views of the potential of the Internet for community building and social change (Turkle 2011, Pullen & Cooper 2010).

The Internet offers new communicative spaces, but it may also limit others. Recent research by Usher and Morrison (2010) suggests that people's growing engagement with new forms of virtual communication and social interaction reveals a migration away from the need for venturing out into 'real' social space. According to these authors, this has the potential to limit the visibility of diversity and the engagement of minority groups in public spaces. It also risks the very real possibility that local community life, and the public sphere more broadly, may become increasingly mainstream. However, Pullen and Cooper (2010) are more optimistic, arguing that the next challenge is to find ways of translating the connections and community generated through global cyberspace into local everyday living spaces so they become more democratic, diverse and embracing of all.

As we noted in Chapter 4, there is also much critical debate in media studies about the limits of social media and the power of 'digital democracy' (Hindman 2009). Public health advocates like Freeman and Chapman (2010, 2007) also express concerns about the ways in which the Internet and social media have been co-opted by advertising, commercial interests and dominant political ideologies (see also chapters 2 and 4). However, community media and social justice advocates such as Curry Jansen et al. (2011) argue that this adds further weight to the pivotal importance of facilitating access to a greater diversity of communicative spaces for individuals, groups and larger communities. This is essential if people are to continue creating new forms of community, and new tactics, for participating in processes of cultural and social change.

CHAPTER SUMMARY

- In this chapter we have stepped aside from traditional, expert-led health communication to explore how people themselves are engaging with community media and online communities in ways that can transform their everyday lives.

- Community and citizens' media exist in the fissures between the public media and commercial media sectors. This third sector, sometimes referred to as 3C media, provides opportunities for citizens to create social dialogue within their communities by telling their own stories, creating their own news and entertainment and sharing these through print, radio, television and online in ways that are not possible in mainstream media.

- Media scholar, Clemencia Rodriguez (2001), has urged us to focus less on what citizens 'do' with their media and more on how participation transforms those citizens and their communities.

- There is now a substantial and growing literature on the effectiveness, strengths and limitations of using community media and online communities for health promotion. In this chapter, we have examined a diverse range of initiatives that mobilise this potential.

- This chapter shows there is much to be gained from building more in-depth understandings about the significance of these communicative spaces in people's lives, and the ways they might be supported, strengthened and sustained.

References

Able Radio 2012, 'Able radio: Focussed on ability'. Accessed 6 May 2014 http://www. ableradio.com/.

Anderson, H. 2012a, *Raising the Civil Dead: Prisoners and Community Radio*, Peter Lang, Bern.

Anderson, H. 2012b, 'Facilitating active citizenship: Participating in prisoners' radio', *Critical Studies in Media Communication*, P.1–15. doi:10.1080/ 15295036.2012.688212.

Australian Institute of Health and Welfare 2011, *The Health of Australia's Prisoners 2010*. Cat. no. PHE 149, AIHW, Canberra.

Best, K. and Butler, S. 2012, 'Disability and communication: A consideration of cross-disability communication and technology', *Disability Studies Quarterly*, 32: 4.

Best, K. and Butler, S. 2014, 'Virtual space: Creating a place for social support in second life', *Space and Culture*, 17: 2. P.1–15. doi: 10.1177/1206331213512235.

Boellstorff, T. 2008, *Coming of Age in Second Life an Anthropologist Explores the Virtually Human*, Princeton University Press, Princeton.

Centers for Disease Control and Prevention (CDC) 2011, *The Health Communicator's Social Media Toolkit*, U.S. Department of Health and Human Services, Atlanta, GA.

Centers for Disease Control and Prevention (CDC) 2012a, *Guide to Writing for Social Media*, U.S. Department of Health and Human Services, Atlanta, GA.

Cole, J., Nolan, J., Seko, Y., Mancuso, K. and Ospina, A. 2011, 'GimpGirl grows up: Women with disabilities rethinking, redefining, and reclaiming community', *New Media & Society*, 13: 1161–1179, first published on 27 April 2011. doi:10.1177/1461444811398032.

Cooper, M. 2010, 'Lesbians who are married to men: Identity, collective stories and the internet online community', in C. Pullen and M. Cooper (eds), *LGBT Identity and Online New Media*, Routledge, New York, 75–86.

Cremorne, L. 2010, 'Murdoch University: ME/CFS support in second life', *The Metaverse Journal*, 31 March 2010. Accessed 6 May 2014 http://www.meta-versejournal.com/2010/03/31/murdoch-university-mecfs-support-in-second-life/.

Curry Jansen, S., Pooley, J. and Taub-Pervizpour, L. 2011, *Media and Social Justice*, Palgrave Macmillan, New York.

Dreher, T. 2010, 'Cultural diversity and the media', in S. Cunningham and G. Turner (eds), *The Media and Communications in Australia*, Allen & Unwin, Crows Nest, 273–284.

Ellis, K. 2008, 'Beyond the Aww factor: Human interest profiles of paralympians and the media navigation of physical difference and social stigma', *Asia Pacific Media Educator*, 19: 23–35.

Forman, A. E., Baker, P., Pater, J. and Smith, K. 2011, 'Beautiful to me: Identity, disability, and gender in virtual environments', *International Journal of E-Politics (IJEP)*, 2 (2): 1–17.

Freeman, B. and Chapman, S. 2007, 'Is YouTube telling or selling you something?', *Tobacco Control*, 16, 207–210. doi: 10.1136/tc.2007.020024.

Freeman, B. and Chapman, S. 2010, 'British American Tobacco on Facebook: undermining article 13 of the global World Health Organization Framework Convention on Tobacco Control', *Tobacco Control*, 19 (3): e1–e9. doi:10.1136/tc.2009.032847

Gillett, J. (2003). 'Media activism and internet use by people with HIV/AIDS'. *Sociology of Health & Illness*, 25(6): 608–624.

GimpGirl 2014, About Us. Accessed 6 May, 2014 www.GimpGirl.com

Gold, J., Pedrana, A., Stoove, M., Chang, S., Howard, S., Asselin, J., Ilic, O., Batrouney, C. and Hellard, M. 2012, 'Developing health Promotion interventions on social networking sites: Recommendations from the FaceSpace project', *Journal of Medical Internet Research*, 14 (1): e30. doi: 10.2196/jmir.1875.

Gorski, D. 2012, 'The perils and pitfalls of "patient-driven" clinical research', *Science-Based Medicine*, July 30, 2012. Accessed 6 May 2014 http://www.sciencebasedmedicine.org/index.php/the-perils-of-patient-driven-clinical-research/.

Hindman, M. 2009, *The Myth of Digital Democracy*, Princeton University Press, Princeton.

Hogg, R. 2002, 'Prisoners and the penal estate in Australia' in D. Brown and M. Wilkie (eds), *Prisoners as Citizens, Human rights in Australian Prisons*, Federation Press, Annandale, 3–20

Holland, K. Blood, W, Pirkis, J. and Dare, A. 2009, Postpsychiatry in the Australian media: The 'vulnerable' talk back', *Asia Pacific Media Educator*, June 2008/July 2009, 19: 143–157.

Howley, K. 2010, *Understanding Community Media*, Sage, Los Angeles.

Katz, V., Matsaganis, M. and Ball-Rokeach, S. 2012, 'Ethnic media as partners for increasing broadband adoption and social inclusion', *Journal of Information Policy*, 2: 279–102.

Laverack, G. 2013, *Health Activism: Foundations and Strategies*, Sage, London.

Lin, W., Song, H. and Ball-Rokeach, S. 2010, 'Localizing the global: Exploring the transnational ties that bind in new immigrant communities', *Journal of Communication*, 60: 205–229.

Meadows, M. and Foxwell, K. 2008, *Community Broadcasting and Mental Illness*, Centre for Public Culture and Ideas, Griffith University, Brisbane.

Miller, N. 2009, 'Spoonfuls of sponsorship making medical students sick', *The Age*, 4 July 2009. Accessed 6 May 2014 http://www.theage.com.au/national/spoonfuls-of-sponsorship-making-medical-students-sick-20090703-d7us.html.

Minc, A., Butler, T. and Gahan, G. 2007, 'The jailbreak health project – Incorporating a unique radio programme for prisoners', *The International Journal of Drug Policy*, 18: 444–446.

Moynihan, R. 2011, 'Power to the people: Could a new informed citizen's movement make medicine healthier?', *British Medical Journal*, 342. doi: 10.1136/bmj.d2002.

Moynihan, R. and Cassells, A. 2005, *Selling Sickness: How the World's Biggest Drug Companies Are Turning Us All into Patients*, Allen & Unwin, Crows Nest.

Moynihan, R., Doust, J. and Henry, D. 2012, 'Preventing overdiagnosis: How to stop harming the Healthy', *BMJ*, 344: e3502. doi: 10.1136/bmj.e3502 (Published 29 May 2012).

National Indigenous Radio Service 2014. Accessed 6 May 2014 http://www.nirs.org.au/.

Outserve 2014, The Association of Actively Serving LGBT Military Personel. Accessed 6 May 2014 http://outserve.org/about/.

Patients Like Me 2013, 'Patients like me: Live better together'. Accessed 6 May 2014 http://www.patientslikeme.com/.

Pedrana, A., Hellard, M., Gold, J., Ata, N., Howard, S., Asselin, J., Ilic, O., Batrouney, C. and Stoove, M. 2013, 'Queer as F**K: Reaching and engaging gay men in sexual health promotion through social networking sites', *Journal of Medical Internet Research*, 15 (2): 1–16.

Pew Research Center 2009, 'The state of the News Media: An annual report on American Journalism', *Pew Research Center Project for Excellence in Journalism*. Accessed 6 May 2014 http://stateofthemedia.org/2009/.

Pew Research Center 2012, 'The state of the news media: An annual report on American Journalism', *Pew Research Center Project for Excellence in Journalism*. Accessed 6 May 2014 http://stateofthemedia.org/2012.

Prison Radio Association 2012. Accessed 6 May 2014 http://www.prisonradioassociation.org.

Prison Radio 2012, 'Mission Statement', *Prison Radio*. Accessed 6 May 2014 http://www.prisonradio.org.

Pullen, C. and Cooper, M. (eds) 2010, *LGBT Identity and Online New Media*, Routledge, New York, 1–11.

Rodriguez, C. 2001, *Fissures in the Mediascape – An International Study of Citizens' Media*, Hampton Press, Cresskill, NJ.

Rodriguez, C. 2010, 'Citizen's media', in J. Downing (ed.), *Encyclopedia of Social Movement Media*, Sage, London, 99–104.

Salazar, J. 2010, 'Digital stories and emerging citizens' media practices by migrant youth in Western Sydney', *3CMedia*, 6 (August): 54–70.

Stewart, S., Hansen, T. and Carey, T. 2010, 'Opportunities for people with disabilities in the virtual world of Second Life', *Rehabilitation Nursing*, 35 (6): 254–259.

Symons, R. 2010, 'Able Radio', *Lias*, Summer 2010, 3–6.

Tsika, N. 2010, 'Compartmentalize your life: Advising army men on RealJock.com', in C. Pullen and M. Cooper (eds), *LGBT Identity and Online New Media*, Routledge, New York, 230–244.

Turkle, S. 2011, *Alone Together: Why We Expect More from Technology and Less from Each Other*, Basic Books, New York.

URLPulse 2012, 'Four walls, no limits: Website measurement and ranking 2012'. Accessed 6 May 2014 http://urlpulse.co/www.fourwallsnolimits.net.

Usher, N. and Morrison, E. 2010, 'The demise of the gay enclave, communication infrastructure theory and the transformation of gay public space', in C. Pullen and M. Cooper (eds), *LGBT Identity and Online New Media*, Routledge, New York, 271–287.

Victorian AIDS Council 2014 Campaigns. Accessed 6 May 2014 http://www.vac.org.au/campaigns

Entertainment-Education: Storytelling and Popular Culture

8

Chapter overview

This chapter provides an introduction to the field of Entertainment-Education (EE). We begin with a brief historical sweep, outlining the origins of EE, its theoretical underpinnings and basic principles. We use a range of practical case studies, from the well-established *Soul City* in South Africa to recent initiatives in Japan, the United States, Nicaragua and the Caribbean, to illustrate the different ways EE is used in communication for health and social change. We also introduce a recent example from Australia focused on sexual health promotion: *Kasa Por Yarn* (KPY), a radio soap series created by young Indigenous people in remote Torres Strait Islander communities. We discuss some of the strengths and limitations of EE, including practical challenges and lessons learned. The chapter concludes by highlighting several interesting trends and emerging issues for EE, including the use of social media and digital games.

Introduction

> A pulsating beat or enticing melody...a story about someone whose life mirrors your own...a truly frank discussion...These are key elements in the mix of ideas that make entertainment-education a powerful, successful communications strategy. When organic characterisation and resonant, familiar scenes mingle with drama and intrigue; when audiences are actively engaged in a learning process; and when stories draw us in because we want to know what people will do, and what will become of them, the opportunity for change is created...
>
> (Population Communication International (PCI) 2003: 12)

Throughout human history, stories have helped us to understand each other and the complexities of our world. Communities and cultures across the globe have used storytelling and performance to strengthen their sense of identity, community and belonging and also to explore social issues and to challenge the politics of the day. Examples such as the Hindu epic stories and dances, Greek myths and legends, Shakespeare's tragedies and comedies, popular cultures of the 1960s and 1970s peace movement, and the resistance music of blues, reggae, hip hop and heavy metal have all been used by cultural groups to say something about who they are, and also as the catalyst for challenge and social change.

We begin this chapter from the position that entertainment is a powerful medium for cultural change. Popular media is enjoyed by people of all backgrounds in almost every corner of the world and it is often the best way to reach people with low literacy, little formal education or income, and those living in marginalised or vulnerable communities. If media is culture-centred, engaging and entertaining, it is popular. And if it is popular, it has a very good chance of making a difference to people's lives.

Entertainment-education in health promotion

Taru: Soap opera for women's health in India

In India, the radio soap opera, *Taru*, was broadcast for a year (2002–2003) in four states, drawing in weekly audiences of ten million people. The story centres around Taru, a young woman who works at the village health centre and is strongly committed to women's issues. With each episode ending with a cliff-hanger, the story follows Taru and her conflicts with various community members as she struggles to initiate changes in people's beliefs and practices. Characters and storylines were designed to generate controversy and conversation about: gender equality, women's empowerment, delayed marriage, small family size, HIV/AIDS prevention and opportunities for breaking down the discriminatory, traditional caste system.

Audiences were intrigued and people everywhere were talking about *Taru*. In just one year, *Taru* achieved a listenership of over 20 million people. Communities became actively engaged with the series through word of mouth promotion by health practitioners. Local villagers organised street performances of episodes. Radio 'listening clubs' in local communities created opportunities for vibrant discussion and the formation of community action groups.

Taru brought about substantial change in promoting gender equality, small family norms and the adoption of contraceptives. In certain villages, condom sales increased by 680% and the sale of birth control pills increased by 580%. Follow-up research after the series showed significantly greater reports of intergenerational dialogue about family planning issues, as well as discussions amongst friends. *Taru* has been followed by a wide range of other EE initiatives across India that now use popular entertainment as a vehicle for bringing communities together and building their capacity for social and cultural change (PCI 2003). For more information about *Taru*, see Singhal (2010).

What is entertainment-education?

In contrast to formal health information and media campaigns, 'entertainment-education' is an approach to health communication that uses the power of popular culture as a tool for change. Health-related themes, stories and scenarios are woven into prime-time television and radio dramas, soaps, reality shows and live performances. Short films, popular music, comics and digital games are also used to share stories, both online and offline. EE aims to generate community conversations about health issues and provide the catalyst for social and political change.

Most contemporary EE includes a multimedia approach supported by community mobilisation strategies. The centrepiece is generally a carefully designed drama, soap opera or reality show series, broadcast through a popular medium. Traditionally, this has been radio or television, but the use of mobile and social media platforms is now commonplace. The style is not formal, didactic or preaching but instead is focused on using the power of storytelling, drama and humour as a conduit for opening up community dialogue about health issues. Multimedia components may include various combinations of supporting print materials (such as booklets, posters or comics), live performance, websites and a range of digital materials (photos, video, music) that are easily shared on social networking sites (SNS).

EE is rarely used as a stand-alone strategy. It is most commonly one part of an integrated, multi-level intervention to achieve social change. The entertainment component is reinforced by a range of strategies that work synergistically to enhance overall effectiveness. Examples can include the following:

- Toll-free helplines and community support services to ensure that audience members have access to support relating to controversial and sensitive personal issues;
- Community engagement opportunities where people can initiate and sustain conversations, create new social networks and participate in social change;
- Publicity strategies, including media news stories, interactive radio talkback segments, public service announcements (PSAs) and paid advertising to engage wider audiences and ensure that issues stay on the public agenda;
- An overarching advocacy strategy to facilitate community mobilising (helping community groups to organise and take action) and direct lobbying of government and other decision-makers (Scheepers et al. 2004).

All components are carefully planned to be mutually supportive over an extended period of time. This might be several months but, in some of the more well-resourced interventions, EE series have continued over decades, such as *Soul City* in South Africa which has been broadcasting since 1992 (see below).

How is EE used in health promotion?

EE has been widely used in contexts where people have low levels of literacy and access to formal education. However, new approaches to EE are rapidly evolving as digital technologies and social media create opportunities for engaging a wide range of audiences. In particular, EE is proving to be an effective way of reaching groups of people unlikely to trust in mainstream education led by experts and 'outsiders', such as marginalised youth (Kawamura & Kohler 2013) and gay men (Pedrana et al. 2013; Gold et al. 2012). EE is especially well-suited for addressing complex health issues where conventional behaviour-change approaches have been relatively unsuccessful, such as sexual health, HIV/AIDS, child abuse, violence against women, and other gender-related issues. It acknowledges that social and cultural change around sensitive issues and/or entrenched practices involves opening up new spaces for conversation and community dialogue. By working through popular culture, EE provides entertaining and non-threatening opportunities for exploring serious issues (see Lacayo & Singhal 2008). The following example provides valuable insights into the ways EE has been used to place complicated and often taboo issues onto the political and public agenda.

EE and human rights

Breakthrough: Music video and multimedia to stop violence against women
According to the UN Development Fund for women (2003 in Lapsansky & Chatterjee 2013), one in every three women in the world will be beaten, raped or otherwise abused during her lifetime. This violence also increases women's vulnerability to other health risks, such as HIV transmission, miscarriage, substance abuse and mental health problems. In the United States and India, the international human rights organisation *Breakthrough* works to promote equality and justice by using EE to open up dialogue about gender-based discrimination, HIV/AIDS, immigrant rights and racial justice.

In 2000, Indian TV audiences were riveted as they watched *Mann ke Manjeere*, a music video featuring a woman working as a truck driver – a housewife who had walked out of an abusive marriage, along with her young daughter, to create a new life. The multi-award winning video placed the issue of domestic violence firmly on the public agenda. As men spoke out in the national media against the culturally entrenched violation of women, the video sparked public discussions everywhere (Lacayo & Singhal 2008).

Following the success of the video, *Breakthrough* developed a suite of multimedia programmes exploring the ways gender discrimination is culturally sanctioned in some parts of India. With over two million women in India infected with HIV/AIDS, *What Kind of Man Are You?* focused on husbands infecting their wives with HIV because they were not willing to wear condoms (Lapsansky & Chatterjee 2013). In the mid-2000s, *Is This Justice?* reached more than 35 million people, changing attitudes and support for women living with HIV/AIDS who were discriminated against by their families (Lacayo & Singhal 2008). In 2009, *Bell Bajao (Ring the Bell)* pushed domestic violence back into the media spotlight with a fresh approach. Instead of focusing on perpetrators, the programme encouraged men and boys everywhere to take responsibility for stopping domestic violence in their communities. The catch-cry, *Ring the Bell,* encouraged men and boys to find non-confrontational ways of interrupting domestic violence by alerting the perpetrator that other men were watching. Sometimes this was as simple as gathering a small group together and 'ringing the doorbell' when they heard violence occurring. *Bel Bajao* used intimate personal storytelling to shift cultural meanings about violence in relationships and to explore possibilities for alternative forms of masculinity (Lapsansky & Chatterjee 2013).

The origins of entertainment-education

The purposeful use of popular entertainment as a strategy for health communication emerged during the mid-1980s. During this period, EE became recognised as a domain of serious scholarship and practice focused on designing and evaluating ways to embed health messages into popular media, to both entertain and educate. In these early years, the aim was to increase audience members' knowledge about educational issues, create favourable attitudes, shift social norms and change behaviour (Singhal & Rogers 1999).

According to Singhal et al. (2012), early EE was strongly influenced by the work of the Mexican television writer–producer–director, Miguel Sabido. Sabido developed a production method for EE soap operas after being inspired by the stunning success of the 1969 television soap opera series, *Simplemente Maria* (Simply Maria) in Peru. The main character, Maria, is a poor young immigrant who moves to the city and is left destitute and alone after her boyfriend discovers she is pregnant. Overcoming innumerable challenges, she finds ways to study, find work and build a new life for herself and her young son.

Maria's story attracted a massive following and mobilised vast numbers of Latin American women to enrol in sewing and literacy classes. Sabido carefully analysed *Simplemente Maria* and used these insights to produce seven highly popular EE 'telenovelas' between 1975 and 1982. These popular television series helped to shift cultural norms, support women and girls' enrolment in literacy classes, encourage the adoption of family planning and promote gender equality (Singhal et al. 2012).

The Sabido method involves creating engaging characters whose lives and stories are both familiar and exceptional. Audiences become emotionally involved as stories unfold and their favourite characters move through journeys of personal change. Social modelling is creatively embedded into the storyline as characters explore the challenges and rewards of adopting new behaviours, such as visiting a health clinic or getting help for a drinking problem. The mix of characters includes some who are:

- positive about change (protagonists);
- resistant to change (antagonists); and
- 'transitional' (people in doubt about the value of doing things differently).

Storylines include dramatic conflicts and complicated social situations requiring characters to make decisions and choices. As the storyline progresses, some transitional characters experiment with new ways of thinking, gradually initiating, refining and practising alternative ways of living their lives. Through this process, storytelling becomes as a way of illuminating pathways to change (Sabido 2004).

For over 25 years, Sabido's pioneering work has provided the springboard for an exponential growth in EE. Currently, there are many hundreds of multimedia EE initiatives in countries around the world, from Africa, South America and Asia to Australia, Japan, the United Kingdom and the United States (see Singhal et al. 2012; PCI 2012, 2013; Singhal & Wang 2009).

EE and international development: Reality television

A broad array of leading international health promotion and development agencies, NGOs and community-based organisations incorporate EE into their work. For example, in many war-torn countries, reality TV is playing an important role in transforming conflict and building peace. In Afghanistan, *Dream and Achieve* is a reality show contributing social renewal by exploring new forms of entrepreneurship. In Guatemala, *Challenge 10: Peace for the Ex* follows former gang members and their personal struggles to live new lives free of crime and violence (Zeilberger 2012).

Reality TV: Transforming conflict in the Congo

In the Democratic Republic of Congo (DRC), a country that has been ravaged by genocide and civil war for the past 30 years, *Tosalel'ango* (Let's Do It!) uses reality TV to help channel young people's frustration and anger into actionable positive change in local communities.

Tosalel'ango stars a local rap artist named Patcha Bay. Congolese youth (18–29) contact the show with an issue they want *Tosalel'ango* to focus on. The producers match two young people with the same issue, and the pair of 'Challengers' is given the opportunity to find a solution. After episodes go to air, viewers email, call and SMS the various ways that they are dealing with similar problems and as a result new problem-solvers spring up.

Watched by 21% of Congolese youth (six million young people), the impact on DRC audiences has been considerable. In 2010, one of the most watched episodes focused on discrimination and the denial of citizenship for children born from mothers raped during war atrocities. Without citizenship, these children were vulnerable to recruitment by armed militia groups as child soldiers. The story generated a massive audience response and provided the catalyst for youth to take action. Working with local lawyers they advocated for reinstatement of citizenship rights for thousands of children incarcerated in orphanages. In another episode, youth Challengers investigated why children of impoverished parents continued to work clandestinely in mines, while their corporate employers were doing little to stop child labour. This episode culminated with the signing of an accord by government officials, mining companies, parents and local NGOs to work together for a more holistic process to prevent child labour in mines.

Later episodes of *Tosalel'ango* focused on Challengers who have been inspired by earlier episodes. With funding from USAID, this ongoing series continues to illuminate new possibilities for Congolese youth to become active participants in peace-building and social change (Okun 2010). *Tosalel'ango* episodes can be found on YouTube and more examples of media for peace-building by the NGO, *Search for Common Ground*, are available at http://www.sfcg.org.

Contemporary EE: Evolution and change

Contemporary EE theories, approaches and technologies

The field of EE has evolved considerably over the past decade. According to Storey and Stood (2013), while early EE focused on changing individual's knowledge, attitudes and behaviours, contemporary approaches tend to include a stronger emphasis on collective responsibility for change. Behaviour change theories still provide an important framework for EE, but the field is now strongly influenced by theories of communication for social change. This incorporates diverse perspectives, such as critical cultural theory (see Chapter 2), and empowerment and critical education theories (see Chapter 7). Narrative theories from the field of media studies are also used to inform the ways in which subversion, shock, humour, sex and emotion are deployed in narrative dramas (see Gesser-Edelsburg & Singhal 2013).

Increasingly, EE interventions are informed by the socio-ecological perspectives that underpin contemporary health promotion. They are designed to achieve change at multiple levels: the individual, communities, organisations and wider society. Mechanisms of change are focused around generating dialogue and public debate, shifting social norms and cultural values and creating supportive environments for change (Scheepers et al. 2004).

Consistent with an ecological approach, EE is expanding its earlier, more specific focus on 'health' to address the wide range of complex human rights, social and environmental issues that contribute to health and illness. Increasingly, EE is being used to help mobilise community advocacy for policy and organisational change focused on protecting rights and challenging unfair, corrupt or discriminatory practices. At a more global level, the growing focus on creating supportive environments for health has seen EE initiatives provide a vitally important catalyst for engaging vulnerable communities with issues of climate change, environmental destruction and protection of biodiversity (PCI Media Impact 2012).

Audiences for EE have also been changing. The earlier focus on 'mass' audiences in developing countries is now complemented by smaller EE initiatives with specific populations and marginalised groups whose members may be widely dispersed across the world. This has largely been possible because of the rapid global expansion of the online environment, mobile digital technologies and social media.

While radio and television are still critical media platforms for EE, interactive and mobile media are also creating a myriad of opportunities for more 'participatory' approaches to EE that involve community members themselves as media-makers, creating their own content, sharing and collaborating together. EE is also finding new ways to tap into the participatory cultures of interactive entertainment, digital gaming and online communities. For readers interested in new EE initiatives in digital gaming and transmedia storytelling, Singhal and Wang (2009) provide a detailed exploration of this field.

Singhal et al. (2012: 323) argue that the trends described above have forged new territory for EE. Accordingly, they propose a contemporary definition of EE as

... a theory-based communication strategy for purposefully embedding educational and social issues in the creation, production, processing, and dissemination process of an entertainment program, in order to achieve desired individual, community, institutional, and societal changes among the intended media user populations.

Soul City institute

The evolution of EE is illustrated in the work of the Soul City Institute for Health and Development Education. Based in South Africa, Soul City Institute is one of the world's most established, well-funded and extensive EE organisations. Established in 1992, when South Africa was on the brink of democratic change, Soul City has focused on a wide range of health and social issues in South African communities. Interventions are based on communication, advocacy and social mobilisation. Soul City's multimedia EE interventions reach 16 million South Africans regularly in nine different South African languages. Many of their programmes have been adapted for other countries around the world. Two most prominent series, *Soul City* and *Soul Buddyz,* include a television series, a radio drama, glossy print materials and a range of community outreach activities. Soul City's programmes also incorporate social media, inviting viewers to comment, share and create their own contributions to aspects of programme development. Links to various blogs and SNS facilitate opportunities for people to exchange advice and information, collaborate and organise local action in their own communities.

Soul City began in 1992 with a serial television drama that has continued over 12, full-length television series for more than 20 years. Early series such as *Soul City IV* created compelling characters and gripping drama interwoven with the inter-related issues of HIV, alcohol and domestic violence. Evaluation research by Scheepers et al. (2004) shows that the series was so popular that it reached 80% of television audiences. Even the actors were deeply affected by the power of the drama, as this public letter from Patrick Molefe Shai illustrates:

> I have been an actor for 27 years, playing a variety of roles with distinctions, and honoured with four Best Actor Awards. When playing an abusive husband in the Soul City IV series, I first-hand experienced the pain and scars I was inflicting on my wife and children.
>
> The events of filming that day are deeply etched in my mind. I was beating my co-actress and as she screamed her face was transformed into my wife's face. Her pleading sounded just like my wife's and the screams of the children actors became those of my children. Mixed emotions swelled inside me. The performance was too real...
>
> I shouted 'Cut!' Then I ran outside and cried. I have never experienced so much pain while performing a character. But this was not just another performance. I had a rare opportunity to see myself in a state of anger. Only this time, I could control my anger. What really pained me that day was the realization that inflicting violence is a choice. When I fought with my wife, bringing her pain and fear, I did not make the right choice. I now know that violence with women is wrong. Thanks to Soul City, today I am a crusader against domestic violence.
>
> Yours truly, for all the victims of domestic violence, Patrick Molefe Shai
> (Usdin et al. 2004: 166)

Soul City IV prompted many emotional private conversations and stimulated wider community dialogue. Communities took action in massive street marches calling for action to address violence against women. In the first five months, over 180,000 men and women called the 'Stop Women Abuse' helpline for crisis counselling. *Soul City IV* also began to impact on the reorientation of services. In partnership with the National Network on Violence Against Women, media publicity was integrated with a national advocacy strategy to influence public debate and lobby government decision-makers. *Soul City IV* helped to facilitate implementation of the Domestic Violence Act; increase availability of critically important support services; and helped people connect with services in their local area. Using popular entertainment as a springboard for change, this multi-level intervention had substantial impacts on individuals, communities and broader society (Scheepers et al. 2004).

Later series, such as *Soul City 11*, explored the lives of people who mobilise their communities and build local community organisations to challenge unfair, corrupt and discriminatory practices. In 2012, work began on developing *Soul City 12* with storylines focused on promoting health and democracy, including the ways communities can act together to improve health and health services. Based on real-life stories, these series explore how communities can organise themselves to become more actively engaged with local government and community decision-making (Soul City Institute 2014).

Soul Buddyz TV series is for 8–14-year-olds. Interwoven into the stories are serious issues which children deal with on a daily basis, including AIDS, relationships, sexuality, bullying, abuse, road safety and other accidents, and the rights of children with disability. *Buddyz Clubs* provides community development through primary schools, educating, enthusing and empowering children to become active agents for change in their own lives and communities.

Other initiatives include *Kwanda*, a 2009 reality TV show in which volunteers work together to build better lives for all. Singhal et al. (2012) describe how communities compete in an 'extreme makeover' competition in order to make their community environments look better and work better. The series follows five communities as they clear streets, garbage dumps and graveyards; establish vegetable gardens for poor people; create services for disabled children; increase children's school attendance; and build profitable businesses around sewing, beading and local cultural products.

Soul City Institute is a world leader in research, development and evaluation of EE and maintains an impressive website of many other EE initiatives. For more information, go to www.soulcity.org.za/.

EE and social movements

Across the world, EE is being used to strengthen social movements by providing the catalyst for media coverage of important social topics and building partnerships with local organisations and coalitions. Drawing on Lacayo and Sinhghal (2008), we will now provide a brief insight into the work of *Puntos de Encuentro* in Nicaragua, one of the most impoverished countries in Central America.

Puntos: Young people in Nicaragua break the silence on sexual diversity
In Nicaragua, the highly successful TV series *Sexto Sentido* (Sixth Sense) was produced by the youth and women's rights organisation, *Puntos de Encuentro* (Meeting Places or Common Ground). With its theme, 'We're different, we're equal', *Sexto Sentido* had the courage to portray lesbian, gay and transgender characters and take on controversial issues in a country whose culture is dominated by the traditional Catholic Church. According to Lacayo and Singhal (2008), the programme managed to avoid being censored and, in fact, captured 70% of the TV-watching audience from 2001 to 2005. Through carefully crafted storylines and characters, *Sexto Sentido* took audiences into the lives of working-class kids as they helped each other deal with homophobia, HIV and racism, as well as breaking the silence around taboo issues of contraception, incest, rape and abortion.

Sexto Sentido is part of a multimedia strategy that includes a daily youth-run radio and Internet talk show, a feminist magazine, billboards, community outreach activities to schools and large-scale distribution of educational audio-visual and print materials. These components work synergistically together to provide young people with 'safe spaces where they can facilitate dialogue and debates to voice opinions, share experiences, challenge biases, negotiate different viewpoints and make decisions about how and where to create change in their lives' (Singhal et al. 2012: 329). These authors emphasise that one of the great strengths of *Puntos* is its combination of entertainment, education and alliance-building partnerships with a range of service providers and local activist organisations. Together, these partnerships are working to support grass-roots social change movements across Nicaragua and Central America.

EE and environmental health justice

Within an ecological model of health, action to address issues such as population growth, climate change and environmental destruction is of pivotal importance. Across the world, loss of biodiversity and environmental damage continue to threaten human livelihoods, food and water supplies and ecological integrity. Communities in resource-poor developing countries are most vulnerable to these effects. One organisation, *PCI Media Impact*, is using EE to assist vulnerable communities in exploring strategies for mitigating these changes and preventing further destruction (PCI 2013; Zeilberger 2012).

In Africa and the Caribbean, EE initiatives are exploring new ways to strengthen local livelihoods while also protecting fragile coastal ecosystems from over-population, environmentally damaging hunting and fishing practices, and resource exploitation. These programmes aim to strengthen social and cultural norms that value the environment and promote conservation and long-term sustainability over short-term interests (PCI Media Impact 2012). We profile a recent programme below.

Radio soap opera Callaloo: Caribbean island nations working together

In the Caribbean, which includes Jamaica, Trinidad and Tobago, St Lucia, the Bahamas, *Callaloo* is a 208-episode radio drama that reaches up to six million people living in 15 island nations. Locally written and produced, the radio drama is part of PCI Media Impact's larger *My Island-My Community* communications programme.

According to USAID,

> The drama follows the lives and loves of four Carribean clans. Characters include a corrupt businessman who plans to drain a wetland, an HIV-positive teen prostitute, a nurse whose philandering boyfriend jeopardises her health, a struggling businessman caught between his work and the environment, and a newspaper editor who takes on environmental issues – and his own father. The show educates listeners about climate change resiliency, biodiversity conservation, and HIV/AIDS while entertaining them with engrossing storylines about betrayal, desire, love and revenge.
>
> (Zeilberger 2012: 29)

Ongoing community discussions about the show and its messages are stimulated through local call-in radio segments and community mobilisation events such as beach clean-up days, tree planting festivals, football matches, cook-off competitions and health testing drives. Initiated in 2012, the comprehensive

My Island-My Community intervention aims to shift social norms around climate change, biodiversity conservation and HIV. Focused on capacity-building, the programme provides training and mentoring to local organisations in each of 15 Caribbean island countries, helping them to establish national coalitions of stakeholder organisations. The aim is to facilitate partnerships within and between countries in the same region and generate collaborative action towards shared goals for health promotion and sustainable environments (PCI Media Impact 2012). More detailed information about these Media for Environment programmes and other EE initiatives can be found at PCI Media Impact www.mediaimpact.org.

This example, along with the earlier case studies, illustrates the diverse applications of EE for health promotion. As the range of issues, audiences and contexts for EE continues to expand, EE practice is evolving rapidly. The next section explores the practical aspects of developing EE programmes.

Principles and practice

Earlier in this chapter, we discussed the Sabido method and how this has informed the way contemporary EE stories are constructed. Human stories can help to bring the hard facts about wider public health and social issues into a more personal context. These issues make much more sense to audiences when they are invited into the intimate spaces of characters' lives as they face challenges, struggle with decisions, take action and find ways to deal with the consequences. In this section, we examine the principles that can be used to guide the overall development of EE programmes.

Scheepers et al. (2004) propose several key principles underpinning effective EE interventions, including:

- Multimedia format
- Multiple reinforcing components
- Drama format sustained over time
- Holistically deals with multiple issues
- Reinforces importance of collectivism
- Theory-based
- Thorough development process, grounded in local contexts and cultures.

'Multimedia format' refers to the combination of radio, television, interactive talk shows, Internet, booklets, education resources which increases the reach of the program. Multiple reinforcing components include entertainment, community mobilising, media publicity and advocacy strategies that work in combination to impact on individuals, communities and wider policy environments.

The drama format is sustained over time because EE recognises that people's perceptions and practices around health don't occur in isolation. Instead, they are shaped by a complicated web of cultural meanings, social relationships and life circumstances. Ongoing engagement with long-running programmes allows characters and storylines to be developed in ways that draw out the complex dimensions of the challenges they encounter.

In contrast to single-issue health promotion campaigns, EE deals with multiple issues. Ongoing storylines provide opportunities for holistic treatment of inter-related issues, such as HIV, culturally entrenched gender relationships, alcohol and violence (see *Soul City IV and Taru*). By reinforcing the importance of collectivism, EE aims to stimulate people's thinking about how they might work together towards change. Collective action enables people to question power relations, shift social norms and challenge unfair power structures. EE can encourage networking, community mobilising and enhancing strategic partnerships between organisations to help build long-term social and political change (Singhal 2013).

Theory-based EE combines theories of behaviour change and social change. Furthermore, EE departs from older communication theories about the effects of media messages on audiences. Instead, it recognises that people are active audiences engaging with media texts in diverse ways that are often quite different from those intended by the producers (see Chapter 2). This means that most contemporary EE takes quite a non-prescriptive route, aiming to influence social and cultural contexts by opening up new conversational spaces where people can discuss the kinds of change they wish to achieve (Singhal et al. 2012). Theories of empowerment and participatory communication are pivotal in EE because they recognise that ordinary people are the key agents of change. As Lacayo and Singhal (2008) note, communication for social change is not about 'telling people what to do', it is about encouraging communities to work together to bring about change for themselves. Successful EE depends on a thorough development process, grounded in local contexts and cultures. This requires extensive formative research and a cyclical, interactive development process that involves community participation in all stages. These stages are briefly outlined in the next section.

Practical steps for developing an EE programme

Most EE programmes are developed through a five-phase process. The following brief guide is adapted from Tufte (2001):

1. **Research and Planning:** Several inter-related issues are selected, based on epidemiological data, expert recommendations and organisational/government health priorities. Formative research is undertaken. This usually involves extensive consultation with various audience groups to help understand the complexity of the issues from their perspectives and to ensure that shows attract and resonate with the target audiences.

2. **Development of the narrative:** Audience research helps to gather personal stories that help the creative teams to develop engaging characters and 'real-life' storylines. Audience members are also actively engaged in script development, pilot-testing and refining the scenes in each episode. A range of service providers, public health and other experts also contribute to the shaping of the key messages and narratives. Phases 1 and 2 may take anything from a few months to several years.

3. **Production:** Most EE interventions engage a professional media production team of writers, artists, actors and specialists to manage the technical aspects of production, broadcast and distribution of multimedia components. However, for organisations on a small budget, EE can still be developed using more simple, low-cost approaches (see below).

4. **Implementation and promotion:** Prior to and during the implementation, community support strategies are put in place. Publicity strategies, including media stories, promotional advertising and public service announcements (PSAs), are used to engage audiences and ensure that issues stay on the public agenda. An overarching advocacy strategy, including community mobilising activities, can be planned in advance but is usually developed in collaboration with audience groups once the programme becomes established.

5. **Evaluation:** This phase involves formative, process and impact evaluation using multiple methods and involving a wide range of stakeholders. The effectiveness of EE processes is commonly measured by:

o   Reach: exposure to the show
o   Recall: of storylines and messages
o   Reception: perceptions of the show's relevance, credibility and quality
o   Resonance: conversations generated about the show and issues.

When a social media component is included, valuable information can also be gathered from user statistics about the level of engagement (page views, 'likes') and interaction between users (comments, sharing, joining blogs and other conversations) (see Gold et al. 2012).

As demonstrated in the earlier example of *Soul City*, impacts can be captured at the level of individuals, communities, organisations and wider policy environments.

Kasa Por Yarn: Talking about sex in remote indigenous communities

In order to illustrate how the above phases work in practice, we will now take a detailed look at a small, low-cost and highly successful EE programme in the Torres Strait Islands and remote, far northern Australia. *Kasa Por Yarn* (KPY) is a multimedia youth sexual health programme implemented *by* and *for* young indigenous people.

Research and planning

In Australia's far north Queensland, remote Aboriginal and Torres Strait Islander (ATSI) communities experience high rates of sexually transmitted infections, with young people aged 15–19 years having a low age of sexual debut, frequent partner change, low sexual health knowledge and very low perception of personal sexual health risk (Fagan & McDonell 2010). Health promotion intervention is challenging as this small population (just over 9,500 people) is dispersed across a vast 48,000 square kilometre in 18 island and 5 mainland communities. Risk is increased because people frequently move between this area, regional Australian cities and nearby Papua New Guinea, where a serious epidemic of HIV/AIDS is well established (PNG National AIDS Council 2010).

Although ATSI people comprise only 2.5% of the Australian population, they represent 83% of the population in this region (ABS 2012). Compared with non-indigenous Australians, ATSI people's life expectancy is approximately ten years less, and self-reports of poor health and high levels of psychological distress are twice that of the general Australian population (ABS 2012).

In 2009/2010, as part of a larger regional sexual health strategy, Queensland Health and *2 Spirits* community organisation facilitated development of *Kasa Por Yarn* (Just for a Chat) targeting young people under 25 and their families. The 12-episode radio drama was aired twice daily through community radio and online for 12 weeks. KPY aimed to encourage community conversations about sexual health and raise awareness of sexual health disadvantage. Produced and broadcast in Yumplatok, a local creole language, the drama takes listeners on a powerful journey through some of the issues affecting lifestyle decisions for local people.

Characters and storylines centre on members of one family as they deal with culturally sensitive issues around HIV/AIDS, teenage pregnancy, safer sex, domestic violence, peer pressure and unwanted sex. The KPY love triangle storyline, for example, explores how young people deal with sexual coercion, teenage pregnancy and infidelity (see Plate 8.1). Local contexts and culture were central to this community-driven project.

Development and production

Development of KPY was participatory and peer-led with the project team being almost entirely local indigenous people. A well-known Torres Strait Islander who had been sexual health worker and now a successful actor and producer took on the pivotal role of community and cultural consultant. He led the community engagement, ensured that storylines were culturally appropriate and relevant, mentored the actors and also played the character of Billy, a local footballer affected by HIV.

A series of community workshops were held in the search for budding local writers, actors, hip hop artists, songwriters and storytellers. In these workshops, local young people developed storylines, provided feedback on scripts and auditioned for parts. Teens, uncles, aunties and parents were all welcome. Approximately 80 local people participated, from project development through to the final broadcast, on steering groups, production teams and as songwriters and musicians. The only non-local participants were the producer, the writer/director and the sound engineer.

Implementation and promotion

Promotion of KPY included a full-page, weekly advertorial in the local newspaper exploring the themes of each episode and featuring a 'Behind the Scenes' interview with one KPY actor or member of the creative team. This generated a buzz around what might happen next in week's episode and gave local young

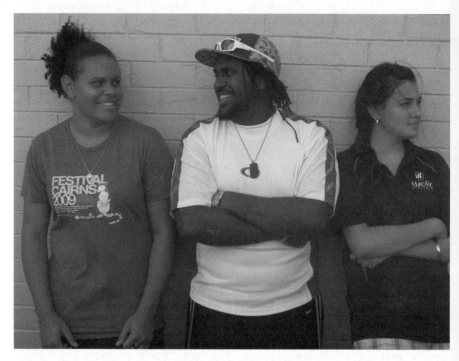

Plate 8.1   Characters in Kasa Por Yarn Series 1: Elise (Rhian Phineasa), J-Dogs (Danny Bani) and Lindy (Talei Elu)

Source: Kasa Por Yarn

people insights into possible career paths and education opportunities. Radio advertisements, posters and community events were used to promote awareness. Social media (YouTube, Facebook, SMS, Twitter, Bebo, WordPress) were used to promote and broadcast the drama, stimulate conversation and provide photos, videos and songs for download. A KPY YouTube channel featured excerpts from episodes, character stories, interviews and music videos.

What KPY achieved

By following the principles of community development and capacity-building, KPY helped to build the confidence and creative skills of local young people, as well as building capacity amongst the wider community for addressing other youth health issues of concern.

Project evaluation

The evaluation measured reach (exposure to the show), recall (of storylines and messages) and resonance (conversation about the drama). The popularity of KPY amongst local people was massive. It reached 84% of the target audience, as direct listeners or indirectly through conversations with others. Almost all listeners (98%) were able to correctly recall storylines or characters and two-thirds spoke about the stories and characters to others. Amongst people who hadn't even heard an episode, one-third were able to talk about the characters and storylines. This provided further evidence of the power of KPY to stimulate community conversations.

Reception, engagement and interaction were substantial given the small population in this region. Over the 12 weeks, Facebook generated 2,245 'friends' and 6,853 Facebook page views. The eight YouTube videos were viewed a total of 2,206 times. Telephone surveys showed that listeners were positive, saying that KPY '[helps people] become more open about the issues' and 'it's OK to talk about these things'. Several negative comments expressed the view that 'it should be taught by parents the right way, not in a public radio show'.

Lessons learned. Focus groups with over a hundred 15–19-year-olds suggested that the storylines could be more engaging for sexually active and single young people. With new information about what worked, what didn't and why, a new series of community workshops began developing *Kasa Por Yarn 2*. Focused on the lives and misadventures of *Alien Krew*, a touring Indigenous youth hip hop band and friends, KPY 2 uses the growing indigenous youth music scene as a vehicle to explore controversial issues. Two community consultants include an award-winning Torres Strait hip hop artist and a well-known community health nurse/radio presenter, who also appear in the series.

Success factors.   Key elements in the success of KPY have been the multimedia approach, robust community consultation and a sound community development approach. KPY created an environment that facilitated healthy community conversations about traditionally sensitive lifestyle decisions and taboo issues. In 2013, the second series was underway, with plans to expand this approach in other indigenous settings across Australia. KPY episodes, videos, music and photos are available at www.kasaporyarn.com. More programme information for both series is at www.kasaporyarn.wordpress.com.

The above profile of KPY is adapted from a case study provided by Dr Patricia Fagan and Heather Robertson, Queensland Health. KPY acknowledges the Torres Strait Island and NPA community members who contributed to and supported KPY.

EE on a small budget: Social media and participatory approaches

As the example of KPY illustrates, the EE process can be easily adapted using simple, low-cost approaches for organisations on a small budget. Low-cost digital cameras, along with mobile and social media, provide a wealth of opportunities for recording and sharing episodes, short clips and other creative content. Kawamura and Kohler (2013) have found that radio drama is often preferred over video because it is more affordable, production is faster and it requires less professional expertise and resources than film or television. Development can be undertaken through workshops in schools and community centres; episodes can be distributed and promoted at no cost through local community radio and online via YouTube and other social media. The authors provide a wealth of practical insights into the processes, challenges and rewards of developing smaller scale radio dramas for media-saturated environments. They provide a detailed profile of two examples, *Body Love* (US) and *Bay for the Seventeen* (Japan), focused on youth sexual health and relationships. Developed and performed *by* and *for* young people, these radio dramas are tailored for small audiences and are their stories are more grounded in local contexts.

Mobile and social media technologies are constantly evolving and this creates a myriad of opportunities for more 'participatory' approaches to EE. The people who were previously considered to be target audiences for EE are increasingly taking on the role of media-makers, sharing experiences and collaborating to create their own content (Pedrana et al. 2013; Gold et al. 2012). As mobile phones, cameras and other digital technologies are becoming more accessible and affordable, audiences are shifting from people 'watching stories about others' to being more active participants in making and sharing their own stories. Many EE programmes now include online competitions inviting audiences to submit their own video or music clips focused on the themes of the show. Not only does this generate greater audience participation, it has also unearthed considerable talent, ideas and inspiration for future programming (Singhal et al. 2012).

Emerging issues and challenges

There is now a growing body of evidence to demonstrate that EE can make a substantial contribution to achieving changes at the level of:

- **Individuals:** knowledge, attitudes, intentions to change behaviours and practices;
- **Communities:** discussion between friends and families, changing community expectations norms, providing support for others to change, community organising and action;
- **Wider society:** access to services, public debate and policy change (Singhal et al. 2012; Lacayo & Singhal 2008; Scheepers et al. 2004).

When change occurs at multiple levels, it is more likely to be maintained over the long term. The sustainability of these changes can also be strengthened by working collaboratively with community organisations and other sectors to influence public policy (see Chapter 10). EE performs well in terms of cost-effectiveness. According to Scheepers et al. (2004), even the relatively high production costs of television and short films are outweighed by the extraordinary capacity of EE to reach a vast proportion of the population, both as direct viewers and, more indirectly, through the wider conversations generated by the programme. EE programmes have excellent 'reach', with audience exposure to shows commonly being around 80% (Singhal et al. 2004). They can also be effectively narrowcast to more specific audiences via community media and SNS (Pedrana et al. 2013). Through their popularity with 'hard to reach' groups, people with low literacy, and those who do not regularly access mainstream print media, EE approaches have an important role in addressing inequities in access to more traditional health promotion interventions.

Key issues

Evaluating the effectiveness of EE continues to be challenging for the field. First, because systemic social change depends on the combined influence of interventions at multiple levels, it is impossible to isolate the entertainment media component and separately measure its 'effects'. Secondly, it is difficult to capture the complexity of social and cultural change processes through conventional evaluation methods (Lacayo & Singhal 2008). As we noted in Chapter 3, social and cultural change is not a simple, linear, 'cause and effect' process. Culture is constantly 'in the making' as people engage with media texts and each other to create meanings around a whole range of cultural practices. Culture is also dynamic and open to continual contestation and change. Cultural change, therefore, is neither highly predictable nor easily controlled or measured. This means that old approaches to evaluating EE, by measuring changes to people's attitudes and behaviour, are not enough to demonstrate the contributions of EE. Useful markers of cultural change need to be identified and indicators are also needed to capture important outcomes, such as social movement building, empowerment and more enabling environments (Freudenberg et al. 2011).

According to Lacayo and Singhal (2008), evaluation in EE should use multiple methods and involve a range of stakeholders. Evaluation should not only reveal *what* changed and *how much,* but also *why and how* that change happened. As well as pre-determined measures of impact, it is important to be flexible enough to capture other important and unexpected outcomes. Evaluation should also include the perspectives of people with different, or even opposing, worldviews in order to understand the full complexity of EE's role in social change processes.

Finally, the importance of building the evidence base for EE interventions cannot be underestimated. While approaches to EE evaluation are continuing to evolve, it is crucially important that innovative EE interventions are well-documented so that success factors can be identified and valuable lessons shared with other practitioners and researchers. From small, local community projects to innovative and highly sophisticated multimedia interventions, evaluation and dissemination of the findings is essential to building the evidence-base to inform future developments.

CHAPTER SUMMARY

- Throughout human history, communities and cultures across the globe have used storytelling and performance to strengthen their sense of identity, community and belonging and also to explore social issues and to challenge the politics of the day.

cont.

- 'Entertainment-education' (EE) uses popular culture, storytelling and other forms of entertainment as a tool for social change. Health-related themes, stories and scenarios are woven into prime-time television and radio dramas, soaps, reality shows and live performances. Short films, popular music, comics and digital games are also used to share stories, both online and offline.

- EE is an effective way of reaching groups of people unlikely to trust in mainstream education led by experts and 'outsiders'. It is especially well-suited for addressing complex health issues, such as sexual health, HIV/AIDS, child abuse, violence against women and other gender-related issues.

- EE acknowledges that social and cultural change around sensitive issues and/or entrenched practices involves opening up new spaces for conversation and community dialogue to provide the catalyst for wider social and political change.

- Entertainment-education is rarely used as a stand-alone strategy. It is most commonly one part of an integrated, multi-level intervention to achieve social change. Most contemporary EE includes a multimedia approach supported by community mobilisation strategies.

- Contemporary EE is a rapidly evolving field. Interactive and mobile media are creating a myriad of opportunities for more 'participatory' approaches to EE with community members as media-makers, creating their own content, sharing and collaborating together.

- Through their popularity with 'hard to reach' groups, people with low literacy and those who do not regularly access mainstream print media, EE approaches have an important role in addressing inequities in access to more traditional health promotion interventions.

References

Australian Bureau of Statistics (ABS) 2012, 'The health and welfare of Australia's aboriginal and Torres Strait islander peoples', *ABS*, Canberra. Accessed 6 May 2014 http://www.abs.gov.au/AUSSTATS/abs@.nsf/lookup/4704.0Chapter100Oct+2010.

Fagan, P. and McDonell, P. 2010, 'Knowledge, attitudes and behaviours in relation to safe sex, Sexually Transmitted Infections (STI) and HIV/AIDS among remote living North Queensland youth', *Australian and New Zealand Journal of Public Health*, 34 (1): 52–56.

Freudenberg, N., Pastor, M. and Israel, B. 2011, 'Strengthening community capacity to participate in making decisions to reduce disproportionate environmental exposures', *American Journal of Public Health*, 101 (1): 123–130.

Gesser-Edelsburg, A. and Singhal, A. 2013, 'Enhancing the persuasive influence of entertajnment-education events: Rhetorical and aesthetic strategies for constructing narratives', *Critical Arts: South-North Cultural and Media Studies*, 27 (1): 56–74.

Gold, J., Pedrana, A., Stoove, M., Chang, S., Howard, S., Asselin, J., Llic, O., Batrouney, C. and Hellard, M. 2012, 'Developing health promotion interventions on social networking sites: Recommendations from the FaceSpace project', *Journal of Medical Internet Research*, 14 (1): 1–17.

Kawamura, Y. and Kohler, C. 2013, 'Applying Sabido's entertainment-education serial drama strategy to serve local radio audiences in the United States and Japan', *Critical Arts: South-North Cultural and Media Studies*, 27 (1): 91–111.

Lacayo, V. and Singhal, A. 2008, *Popular Culture with a Purpose! Using Edutainment Media for Social Change*, Oxfam-Novib, Den Haag, Netherlands.

Lapsansky, C. and Chatterjee, J. 2013, 'Masculinity matters: Using entertainment education to engage men in ending domestic violence in India', *Critical Arts: South-North Cultural and Media Studies*, 27 (1): 36–55.

Okun, R. 2010, 'Focus on DRC: The real world Congo', *Search for Common Ground*. Accessed 6 May 2014 http://thecommongroundblog.com/2010/12/16/focus-on-drc-the-real-world-congo.

Papua New Guinea National AIDS Council 2010, 'Papua New Guinea HIV prevalence: 2009 Estimates'. Accessed 6 May 2014 http://aid.dfat.gov.au/HotTopics/Documents/2009pnghivprevalence.pdf.

Pedrana, A., Hellard, M., Gold, J., Ata, N., Howard, S., Asselin, J., Ilic, O., Batrouney, C. and Stoove, M. 2013, 'Queer as F**K: Reaching and engaging gay men in sexual health promotion through social networking sites', *Journal of Medical Internet Research*, 15 (2): 1–16.

Population Communication International 2003, 'Entertainment, education, empowerment: Annual report 2003', *PCI*, New York. Accessed 6 May 2014 http://mediaimpact.org/.

Population Communication International – Media Impact 2012, 'Callaloo: My Island, My Community: Annual Report 2011', *PCI*, New York, Accessed 6 May 2014 http://mediaimpact.org/.

Population Communication International – Media Impact 2013, 'Annual Report 2012', *PCI*, New York. Accessed 6 May 2014 http://mediaimpact.org/.

Sabido, M. 2004, 'The origins of entertainment-education', in A. Singhal, M. J. Cody, E. M. Rogers and M. Sabido (eds), *Entertainment-Education and Social Change: History, Research and Practice*, Eribaum, Mahwah, New Jersey, 61–74.

Scheepers, E., Christofides, N., Goldstein, S., Usdin, S., Patel, D. and Japhet, G. 2004, 'Evaluating health communication – A holistic overview of the impact of soul City IV', *Health Promotion Journal of Australia*, 15 (2): 121–133.

Singhal, A. 2010, *Riding High on Taru Fever: Entertainment-Education Broadcasts, Ground Mobilization, and Service Delivery in Rural India*, Entertainment-Education and Social Change Wisdom Series, OxfamNovib, Netherlands.

Singhal, A. 2013, 'Fairy Tales to digital games: The rising tide of entertainment education', *Critical Arts: South-North Cultural and Media Studies*, 27 (1): 1–8.

Singhal, A., Cody, M. K., Rogers, E. M. and Sabido, M. (eds) 2004, *Entertainment-Education and Social Change: History, Research, and Practice*, Lawrence Erlbaum Associates Publishers, Mahwah, NJ.

Singhal, A. and Rogers, E. 1999, *Entertainment-Education: A Communication Strategy for Social Change*, Erlbaum, Mahwah, NJ.

Singhal, A. and Wang, H. 2009, 'Entertainment-education through digital games', in U. Ritterfeld, M. J. Cody and P. Vorderer (eds), *Serious Games: Mechanism and Effects*, Routledge, New York, 271–292.

Singhal, A., Wang, H. and Rogers, E. 2012, 'The rising tide of entertainment-education in communication campaigns', in R. E. Rice and C. K. Atkin (eds), *Public Communication Campaigns*, 4th Edition, Sage, Beverley Hills, CA, 323–335.

Soul City Institute (2014) 'Soul City Institute for Health and Development Education'. Accessed 6 May 2014 www.soulcity.org.za/

Storey, D. and Stood, S. 2013, 'Increasing equity, affirming the power of narrative and expanding dialogue: The evolution of entertainment education over two decades', *Critical Arts: South-North Cultural and Media Studies*, 27 (1): 9–35.

Usdin, S., Singhal, A., Shongwe, T., Goldstein, S. and Shabalala, A. 2004, 'No short cuts in entertainment-education: Designing soul City step-by-step', in A. Singhal, M. J. Cody, E. M. Rogers and M. Sabido (eds), *Entertainment-Education and Social Change: History, Research, and Practice*, Lawrence Erlbaum Associates, Mahwah, NJ, 153–176.

Zeilberger, C. 2012, 'Development with a side of drama', *US Agency for International Development*, NW, US. Accessed 6 May 2014 http://www.usaid.gov/global-waters/december-2012/development-with-drama.

Health Activism: Community Action for Change

9

Chapter overview

This chapter explores the role of health activism in communication for health. It explains the importance of working *with* communities to strengthen their capacity to take collective action for social and political change. We examine the principles and practice of health activism, why they are important and how activism can be used as a powerful communication tool for public health. We discuss a range of case studies to provide practical insights and to illustrate some of the challenges and lessons learned. This chapter begins with three recent examples of health activism to set the scene for the discussions that follow.

Introduction: Three activist campaigns

The 'Tell Kelly Clarkson to drop tobacco sponsorship' campaign

Tobacco sponsorship of live music and events targeting teens and children has been banned in many countries. However, in Indonesia enforcement of tobacco control measures is almost non-existent, and big tobacco companies voraciously pursue the recruitment of young smokers. Sponsored festivals, music concerts and free live events are saturated with tobacco advertising and roving teams of Indonesian youth offering cigarette give-aways, tobacco packs, competitions and sign-ups to kids as young as eight (Lewis & Lewis 2009). So when anti-tobacco activists heard that Kelly Clarkson's 2010 Indonesia concert was sponsored by PT Darum, Indonesia's third largest tobacco company, they swung into action. The singer had sold over 20 million albums since winning the US talent show, American Idol, in 2002. Her music deals with themes of heartbreak, independence and self-empowerment for women and young teens. Ironically, this made her the ideal target for direct action against tobacco industry sponsorship of live music and events for teens and children.

Supported by a range of anti-tobacco and child welfare agencies in Indonesia, the *Campaign for Tobacco-Free Kids* wrote to Clarkson's management requesting that the sponsorship be withdrawn. After no response was received, a group of young activists in Australia set up an open Facebook page called 'Tell Kelly Clarkson to Drop Tobacco Sponsorship'. In less than a week, the site had 450 members, many of whom also posted on Clarkson's fan page asking her to drop the sponsorship. As the pressure from her fans rapidly escalated, the singer publicly defended herself on her personal blog. The public tussle between a celebrity and her fans attracted substantial press coverage and created a public relations nightmare for the star.

A few days later, Clarkson and her management announced that the sponsorship deal had been withdrawn. The Indonesian concert went ahead – with Clarkson but without the tobacco industry. Several months later, another tobacco-sponsored Indonesian international music festival faced unprecedented levels of protest. This time, thousands of activists took action. They signed online petitions, commented on tweets and posted on the fan blogs and Facebook accounts of headline band members from the United Kingdom, the United States and Australia. This activity sparked a vitriolic UK media campaign condemning the involvement of Welsh band, Stereophonics. Controversially, the US band Neon Trees agreed to donate their entire appearance fee to an Indonesian cancer charity. In Australia, Wolfmother reconsidered their appearance and refused to be part of the festival the following year. Pressure from activists had successfully forced these internationally acclaimed artists, their management and promoters to acknowledge the issue and reconsider their future association with tobacco sponsorship (Hefler et al. 2013).

Saudi Women2Drive

The Muslim kingdom of Saudi Arabia has a poor record of protecting women's human rights (Human Rights Watch 2013). Forced detention, rape and violence against women are illegal, but many cases have received pitifully light disciplinary measures. It is also against the law for women to drive a vehicle of any kind. Numerous Saudi women have been sentenced to prison for driving unlawfully on the grounds of challenging their husband's authority and violating a religious decree. In 2013, Wajeha Al-Huwaider was arrested after she drove across the city with supplies in response to a call for help on Twitter from another woman who had been left for a week, locked in a family compound by her husband and was running dangerously low on food and water (Pollitt 2013).

The Saudi women's activist movement, *Women2Drive*, has been working for change since 2011 when human rights campaigner Manal al-Sharif was jailed for posting an online YouTube video of herself driving. Since then, Saudi women have continued to upload driving videos, some of them taken by husbands supporting their cause. As videos are taken down by authorities, they are soon replaced by others. These women activists are strategically using the global forum of the Internet to raise awareness and generate support for changes to laws which they believe are threatening women's health and endangering their lives.

In rural communities, citizen activists are also taking action to undermine the laws, with men secretly teaching their daughters to drive and women driving in disguise or dressed as men (Toumi 2013). In late 2013, when Saudi Prince Alwaleed bin Talal publicly announced his support for changing the laws, the *Women2Drive* movement recorded this as a small but significant step forward (Al Jazeera 2013).

Highways, health and human rights: Colombian women's sex strike

Barbacoas is an isolated agricultural town in Colombia, South America. In 2011, there was only one highway connecting the town to the rest of the country, and the poor state of this unpaved road meant that the 57-kilometre route took ten hours. The local government had not addressed community concerns about the road for 18 years, even though the situation had prevented the delivery of critical supplies to the town. In 2011, after a 23-year-old woman died while giving birth on the highway because the ambulance could not reach the hospital in time, local women organised themselves in a unique form of protest known as 'lysistratic non-action'.

Campaigners claimed that government inaction was a human rights issue and that sex had to be banned because it was unethical to bring children into the world if the town did not offer basic rights to survive. With the slogan, 'No more sex. We want our road', women announced the start of the 'crossed legs movement'. Almost 300 women participated, including the wife of the mayor of Barbacaos. Men added weight to the campaign by going on hunger strike. After four months, the pressure on powerful men in the community became too much. On 11 October 2011, authorities finally initiated work on construction of the new road. The municipal mayor, emboldened by his wife's political courage, also managed to persuade the country's transport minister to pledge US$21 million to pave the first 27 kilometre of the road. At the official opening of the highway, both of these men lauded the success of the campaign (Liu 2011).

What is activism?

As each of the above case studies illustrates, activism is about citizens and communities taking action for social and political change. Activism can involve small acts of resistance by individuals, such as signing an online petition, boycotting a product or prompting others to think more critically about their living and working conditions. Activism is also widely used by communities seeking to defend local assets (such as a school threatened with closure, an unpolluted water supply, or a pristine ecological area) or to secure much-needed resources to improve health and community cohesion (such as a safer road, improved public transport, or a new community centre). At the other end of the spectrum, activism can involve many thousands of people whose actions are linked together through large, international activist organisations (such as Greenpeace), and also through broader, long-term social movements, including the human rights, environmental, HIV/AIDS and women's health movements. Activism, therefore, can be undertaken at many levels from the local to the global.

Activism can be understood as a 'process by which groups of people exert pressure on organisations, employers and other institutions to change policies, practices or conditions that the activists find problematic' (Reber & Kim 2006: 316). Activism is also action on behalf of a cause. It can be distinguished from other forms of advocacy for public health because it involves 'action that goes beyond what is conventional or routine, relative to the actions of others in society' (Laverack 2013). What this means is that, instead of working through conventional avenues, activism uses unconventional, direct actions to draw attention to injustice and create the stimulus for change.

The strategies needed to achieve these goals vary between countries and contexts, depending on laws, cultural norms and values. As the above case study illustrates, in Saudi Arabia, action that would go unnoticed in most other countries, such as a woman driving the family car, is treated as an unconventional act of civil disobedience. It is also considered to be a subversive expression of political protest in support of the wider struggle for women's human rights in that country.

Clearly then, activism has different forms and meanings depending on the context and the people using it. Nonetheless, the central focus of activism is to educate, alert, inspire and eventually involve a large proportion of the community in taking some kind of collective action to put pressure on decision-makers (Ricketts 2012). Community activism aims to intensify this pressure by raising awareness amongst people not previously engaged with this issue and building a social movement – a critical mass of citizens who are committed to the cause (Freudenberg et al. 2009).

Activism commonly involves people doing, or refusing to do, certain things, and often in ways that are outside the bounds of accepted cultural, gender and social expectations, or which break rules, regulations or the law (Lakey 2011a).

- People may *do* something they normally would *not* do. For example, writing letters to the newspaper, participating in protest rallies, stunts and events; vigils, picketing, sabotage of important events and shareholder meetings; online activism (such as email bombing, virtual sit-ins and culture jamming); creating protest art, music or graffiti; community education and consciousness-raising, lobbying or instigating legal action.
- People may *stop* doing what they normally *would* do. For example, strikes, stopworks and work slowdowns; sanctions and boycotts, refusing to pay taxes or fines, lysistratic non-action (sex strike), refusing to wear religious symbols, uniforms and/or certain clothes.

Health activism

While there are many definitions, Laverack (2013: 137) defines health activism as 'action that involves a challenge to the existing order whenever it is perceived to influence people's health negatively or has led to an injustice or an inequality'. It involves a range of tactics that go beyond the conventional or routine in order to 'redress the imbalance of power that has created the situation in the first place'.

Health activism and social movements for health have a very important influence on our healthcare systems and are a major force for change in larger society (Brown et al. 2004). Health activism is often focused on specific health-related issues, such as access to health care, or the needs of people with particular disease or disability. The actions of health activists in many countries have achieved significant influence over important healthcare reforms, recognition of patients' rights, improved safety of pharmaceutical drugs and medical treatments, as well as more equitable and accessible health care for women, ethnic minorities, disadvantaged communities and marginalised groups (Zoller 2005).

Broader social movements, such as the women's health movement, the AIDS movement and disability rights movement, have worked tirelessly over many decades to challenge existing scientific and medical knowledge by providing alternative accounts of people's experiences with medications, treatments and health care. These health activists have ensured that the perspectives of everyday citizens are considered as legitimate evidence used to inform expert decision-making processes. Their actions have been pivotal in successfully altering many medication and treatment forms (e.g. mental health), achieving greater recognition for non-medical therapies and changing the way clinical trials are conducted (e.g. HIV/AIDS) (Brown & Zavestoski 2004).

Beyond the health system, health activism also plays a vitally important role in generating changes to the wider social, political and environmental factors that influence people's health, including those that perpetuate social injustice and health inequity. For example, in 2013, disability pressure groups in Australia achieved success in their four year campaign for a National Disability Insurance Scheme to reduce inequities in access to health care, secure housing, training and employment for people living with disability (Every Australian Counts 2013). At the same time, disability groups in the United Kingdom were organising widespread activism in opposition to the conservative Cameron government's proposed amendments to the Welfare Reform Act that would see dramatic cuts to services and social protection measures for people affected by disability (Hardest Hit Coalition 2013).

Activism has also enabled broader health social movements to maintain the momentum of long-term campaigns by refocusing public attention on long-term struggles for change. For example, the environmental breast cancer movement has significantly increased public and scientific awareness of the environmental causes of breast cancer in women's homes and workplaces, helping to bring about tighter controls over the pesticides and chemical industries (Brown and Zavestoski 2004; Brown et al. 2004).

These examples illustrate the ways in which activism is used by everyday citizens to hold institutions, governments and corporations accountable for their decisions, as well as to agitate for action to address important social issues that affect their lives. Health activism, therefore, is a strategy that involves disrupting the usual activities of the powerful to ensure that ordinary people, including those without great financial resources or political leverage, have a political voice on matters that affect health.

Foundations of health activism

Origins of health activism: From sanitation to social justice

Health activism has a formidable history. Over centuries, health reformers have collaborated with pressure groups and social activists to focus public attention on the causes and solutions for many public health problems. As early as the mid-1800s, the UK public health reformer Edwin Chadwick (1800–1890) met with local pressure groups regarding their concerns about growing urbanisation, contaminated water supplies and the desperate need for better sanitation for people living in the poorest areas of London. At around the same time, local doctor John Snow (1813–1858) was also deeply troubled by the recurring cholera outbreaks devastating these communities. Snow went into the Soho district, asking people about their health in order to map the distribution of disease. His research provided empirical evidence that located the source of the problem: contaminated water supplies from the 'Broad Street pump'. The private water supply company responsible for the pump had been cutting costs by drawing dirty water from the nearby, but most polluted, parts of the river where sewage was discharged.

The combined work of Snow and Chadwick had a radical impact on public thinking about the relationship between people's living and working conditions, and their risk of disease. This unconventional alliance between scientific experts and concerned citizens' groups generated vibrant public debate which influenced the thinking of other professionals about the need for change. Collectively, they lobbied decision-makers and government. Their combined actions, heavily publicised in the newspapers of the time, led to the landmark development of the first government Public Health Act (1948) which provided the framework for London's first coordinated response to sanitation, safe water supplies and a range of other problems faced by the city's poorest people (Crossier 2012; Snow 1999).

During the mid-1800s to mid-1900s, there was a marked increase in organised efforts to rally public opinion against social injustice. In the United Kingdom, the United States, Europe and many colonised countries around the world, activism played a crucially important role in abolishing slavery, achieving women's right to vote and raising awareness about discrimination based on race, ethnicity and social class. At around the same time, there was a revolutionary shift towards industrial production of machines and material goods. The working poor, including young children, were concentrated in factories, mines and small-scale workhouses, often under appalling conditions. In England and France, concepts of 'labour justice' emerged in response to public concerns about the unfair distribution of income and wealth between owners of capital and workers. Workers began to organise themselves to form trade unions so they had more power to negotiate with employers. These early activists achieved landmark advances towards safe working conditions, fair wages, protection for injured workers and their families and actions to prevent environmental contamination in local communities (Curry Jansen et al. 2011).

Throughout the 1960s and 1970s, activists in many countries used mass protests, civil disobedience and other disruptive actions to challenge the existing order and structures of power in society. The US civil rights movement achieved huge advances in the rights of African-Americans. The feminist movement established itself as a powerful force for the emancipation of women, demanding access to the contraceptive pill, reproductive choice and new steps towards gender equality in education, work and domestic life. The empowerment of women and minority groups also facilitated a more participatory public sphere – with a more diverse array of individuals and groups becoming actively engaged in public activities designed to change the way society functioned. This pressure on governments led to stronger commitments to providing social safety nets for the disadvantaged and more equitable opportunities for education, employment, housing and health care.

The expansion of global capitalism in the 1980s and 1990s brought new economic and political conditions of rapid growth and the deregulation of workplaces and financial institutions by neoliberal governments in the United Kingdom, the United States, Europe and Australia who believed they should not interfere with the workings of free markets. However, the economic benefits of this period were concentrated with a small proportion of the population, and income inequalities substantially increased. By 2010, the income gap between the very rich and the 'other 99%' of the world's population had dramatically increased, with income inequality in the United States reaching the worst seen since the Great Depression of 1928 (Wilkinson & Picket 2010).

Over this period, governments in many countries, and particularly the United Kingdom and parts of Europe, have tightened spending on infrastructure for health and education and removed many social protection measures (Nathanson & Hopper 2010). At the same time, massive global corporations have reported multi-billion dollar profits. Globally, inequalities in access to resources, jobs, affordable housing and health care have continued to widen dramatically – both within and between countries. This uneven distribution of resources and power has contributed to growing health inequalities and continues to have the greatest impact on those lower down the social gradient (Laverack 2012).

According to the Marmot Review (2010), health inequities are produced by social norms, policies and practices that tolerate, or actually promote, unfair distribution of and access to power, wealth and other necessary social resources. This affects the way people live, their consequent chances of illness and their risk of premature death. Laverack (2013) argues that, within this context, public health and health promotion practitioners have an important role in engaging with activist groups to address the causes of social injustice and health inequalities.

Activism in contemporary health promotion

Activism and community action are effective approaches for empowering people to engage in collective efforts that are directed towards increasing community control over the determinants of their health (WHO 1998). 'Strengthening community action' is a key action area of the WHO Ottawa Charter for Health Promotion (1986). Strengthening the capacity of local people in the context of their communities, and the government and other institutions that support those communities, is a principle of the Alma Ata Declaration for Primary Health Care (1978) and recent concepts of primary health care (WHO 2008).

Activism is an upstream approach to health promotion that moves beyond a focus on individual change to influence change at the level of communities, organisations and wider society. As a health promotion strategy, it leads to more sustainable change through its focus on community empowerment and capacity building (Laverack 2013). While community activism can work as a stand-alone strategy, it is more likely to achieve longer-term change when combined with formal public health advocacy efforts to change corporate practices and influence healthy public policy. Activism, therefore, is most effective when used as one element of a comprehensive, integrated, multi-level mix of health promotion interventions.

Strengths and limitations

Activism generated by communities themselves can complement and strengthen other health promotion strategies, particularly the more formal processes of advocacy to influence healthy public policy. In contrast to public health *advocacy*, in which groups tend to work 'within the existing system', health *activism* commonly operates outside the bounds of institutionalised political channels (Brown et al. 2004). It has a key role in mobilising strong public support for the policy changes being sought through formal public health advocacy processes, thereby increasing their effectiveness and sustainability.

Activism has several important roles in 'building healthy public policy' (WHO 1986). First, by raising awareness, influencing public opinion, building support for change and generating community action to pressure decision-makers. Second, activism builds the capacity of ordinary people to become active participants in community decision-making and to have an influence on wider policy processes.

Activism and healthy public policy

Activists can influence the policy-making cycle at several stages. First, by bringing issues onto the public agenda, including unrecognised health issues or those being strategically 'overlooked' by decision-makers. As part of the policy-making process, community activist groups often respond to calls for public comment on draft policies before they are implemented. During the implementation phase, they gather information about the effects of the policy on their communities (sometimes referred to as 'lay epidemiology'). At the review stage, activist groups commonly pressure decision-makers by publicising this information as evidence to support the need for amendments to the policy (Brown et al. 2004).

An example is 'Gulf War Syndrome', a condition experienced by a large proportion of people returning from active military service. It remained largely hidden until patient activists placed the spotlight on governments' responsibility to recognise and provide care for its veterans. More recently, following the invasions of Iraq and Afghanistan, policies relating to support for veterans have been reviewed in response to activist groups of veterans and their families.

Health practitioners should have a good understanding of the theoretical and practical importance of activism so they are better able to support individuals, pressure groups and communities seeking to use this approach for taking more control over the decisions and resources that affect their lives (and health).

Theoretical perspectives and models

Activism has been studied by multiple disciplines, including history, law and political studies, education, community development and media studies – all of which share a common interest in understanding the dynamics of social change. The work of health activism scholars and practitioners is informed by the theoretical perspectives of cultural studies, post-colonialism, feminism and subaltern studies (Dutta 2011). These theories have a particular focus on issues of culture and identity, marginalisation, power and resistance – and they are often deployed by researchers and practitioners who are interested in challenging socially structured inequalities.

Health activism is underpinned by the idea that educated, empowered and organised groups of citizens have an important role in creating healthy social change (Laverack 2013: 93). It is guided by values of social justice, equity and community empowerment. Health activism aims to address broader social and political agendas for health by focusing on the structural and systemic causes of health inequities. It aims to challenge the existing social order by disrupting the usual flows of power between dominant groups (power-holders) and the communities and people with less power, resources and access to institutional channels of political influence.

Before we explore how activism works in practice, we will briefly outline three key theoretical concepts that help us to better understand the principles of effective activism. These include: critical consciousness, radical activism and democratic practice.

Critical consciousness: Education model

Activism aims to mobilise people by raising 'critical consciousness'. This concept draws on the work of the Brazilian educator, Paulo Freire (1921–1997), who believed that people and communities can only overcome powerlessness, oppression and inequity by developing their ability to think critically about the factors influencing their lives (Minkler & Wallerstein 2010). As communities come to understand how their circumstances are related to underlying social and political causes, they are better positioned to develop solutions and strategies for change. Critical consciousness is an important element of activism because it helps to facilitate people's sense of empowerment to bring about change. Most of the work of activist groups involves communication with a range of audiences to raise awareness about an issue in ways that specifically aim to build people's critical consciousness.

Radical activism: Conflict model

Radical activism is one approach used by less powerful groups to influence decision-makers. In his book, *Rules for Radicals* (1971), the US civil rights activist Saul Alinsky (1909–1972) argued that agitation to the point of conflict is a necessary prerequisite for change. For Alinsky, change meant movement and that movement invariably created friction. Much of his work was with poor African-American communities of Chicago in the 1930s, helping them to organise strong community action groups to confront local politicians about problems of overcrowded schools and poor housing in the troubled 'Back of the Yards' communities.

Alinsky believed that confrontation pushes tension to the brink of conflict and this provides important opportunities for less powerful people to experience their own authority to challenge the powerful. Conflict also attracts media attention and forces social problems into the public arena. While there are many critiques of radical activism (see Derville 2005), Alinsky claimed that a radical approach creates the conditions for communities to leverage their power and political influence on decision-makers (English 2007).

Participatory democracy: Active citizenship model

In contrast to the radical approach, activism can also be understood as an essential component of a healthy democratic society. According to lawyer and community activist Aidan Ricketts (2012: 6), 'activism, social change advocacy and democracy are inextricably linked. It is the work of activists and social movements which pushes society along, prompts it to deal with its own failing and inequalities and helps to manifest a vision of a better world.' Activism provides opportunities for citizens to take an active role in the affairs of the community and to be prepared to make those concerns heard. In doing so, activism aims to exert influence within democratic processes.

Democracy is a contested term that is theorised and practised in many different ways. Generally though, democracy is based on 'the premise that political power derives from the will, or at least the consent, of the people' (Ricketts 2012: 6). Elected government representatives closely monitor the views of the people (public opinion) as they carry out their roles as legislators and custodians of democracy because ultimately they depend on public approval to remain in office. Corporations (such as alcohol or pharmaceutical companies) and institutions (such as religious organisations) are also highly sensitive to public opinion to ensure they maintain markets for their products, shareholders, members and supporters. What this means is that ordinary citizens, acting collectively, can have considerable power to influence their policies and practices.

Participatory democracy involves people taking an active role in public activities designed to influence the way governments, corporations and other institutions function. At its most basic, this involves people exercising their right to vote in elections, but it also refers to more vibrant cultures of political participation mediated through music and art, graffiti, video-making, citizen journalism, protest, assembly, lobbying, strikes and legal action. Activism and social movements aim to moderate the way in which power is exercised in society by increasing opportunities for citizens to actively influence decision-making. As a form of democratic practice, activism is pivotal in building and maintaining a healthful and democratic society (Ricketts 2012; Lewis 2008).

Principles of effective activism

Over history, people have used activism when other options are less available to them – or when other conventional strategies have not been effective. While activism has traditionally been used by oppressed or marginalised groups with less power to participate in public decision-making, contemporary health activists come from all walks of life and are united by their common concern for challenging the dominance of powerful social groups that contribute to social injustices and health inequalities.

Three principles of effective health activism include: empowerment and participation, collective action through community organising and a commitment to non-violence.

Principle 1: Empowerment and participation

Empowerment is a process by which people and communities are supported in a process of gaining more control over the decisions and resources that affect their lives. As Laverack (2013: 7) notes, 'there are many situations in which people are prevented from living a healthy lifestyle because of the lack of opportunity or an injustice'... 'People may be sure about what they want, but are often less certain about the means to achieve it, especially how to gain access to political influence and resources'. For this reason, most activist organisations have a strong focus on helping people to develop the confidence, knowledge and skills so they can take a more active role in community decision-making. This includes getting issues onto the public agenda and putting pressure on decision-makers whose policies or practices affect them adversely (Keleher 2011).

Women's activism, for example, has over many decades brought women together through networks of individuals and groups to share knowledge and learn about tactics and communication skills for achieving social change. Many activist groups provide resource kits and training opportunities for members and supporters. Topics include running meetings, conflict resolution, fund-raising, media relations and speaking to the mass media, scientific debate and skills for lobbying, as well as understanding activist's rights and strategies for protecting their privacy and safety. Several recent books and online resources provide useful practical guidelines and tips for strategic mapping of campaigns, networking and effectively managing people, mobilising funding and other resources (Shaw 2013; Fitzroy Legal Service 2013; Ricketts 2012; The Change Agency n.d.).

Video activism, women's empowerment and media-making

See it, film it, change it!
In recent years, health activism has also focused on facilitating opportunities for people to actively participate in 'media-making' as a way of representing their perspectives and becoming agents of community change. Using low-cost, simple digital tools, individuals and communities are creating a diversity of images, video, audio, graphics and text that are easily uploaded, shared and networked via the Internet. Marginalised groups are also becoming more actively engaged in 'talking back' to mainstream media, challenging mainstream representations and speaking up about issues in their communities (Anderson 2012; Holland et al. 2009). One approach, video activism, is emerging as a pivotal tool for activists with low education and literacy levels and those with little access to formal channels of communication and political influence.

In poor villages across India, community media programmes run by *Video Volunteers* have facilitated women's empowerment as agents of change even though many can neither read nor write. Community video units provide access to video skills training, equipment, workshops on basic spoken-word reporting and story-building. These women become part of a network of community correspondents who make three-to-four-minute videos that address pressing issues and local concerns. Topics have included rape, family violence, honour killings, child marriage, lack of sanitation and girls' access to education and contamination of local water supplies. Videos are screened to local audiences at community gatherings, religious groups and school settings to raise awareness and generate community action towards local solutions. The videos are strategically used to lobby local decision-makers and politicians.

Through the *India Unheard* network, women's stories are distributed more widely to national and global audiences via YouTube, social media sites and online community media stations, such as BlipTV. Community-produced news content is fed to international media outlets, achieving important coverage in mainstream media. Through video activism, women in some of India's most marginalised communities are becoming highly valued citizen journalists exposing under-reported issues and mobilising community action to address poverty, discrimination and social injustice (Video Volunteers 2013).

Principle 2. Community organising and collective action

While individual activists can achieve a great deal, the most effective way to bring about social change is through organised groups of people working collectively to address an issue they feel strongly about. Communities and groups need to organise themselves so they can access the resources, skills and capacities to have the level of influence needed to bring about social change.

Even small community groups with limited resources need to establish structure, strong leadership and the ability to better organise their members so they can survive long enough to achieve the changes they want for their communities. According to Laverack (2013: 95), 'by operating collectively, activists can also gain several advantages. They can undertake larger tasks, such as organising a national campaign, can benefit from sharing roles and responsibilities and can also give a feeling of solidarity and mutual support to one another'.

One of the most effective ways to build capacity for influence is to collaborate with others through partnerships with existing community organisations and pressure groups with mutual interests. Pressure groups aim to create a sustained political presence that maintains pressure on decision-makers around specific issues, such as disability rights, the needs of single parents, or environmental protection. Small activist groups can also gain greater political influence by working collectively through larger networks, alliances and coalitions, including trade unions, health professional alliances, consumer health groups and patient networks involving active groups of patients, their supporters and volunteers. In the following case study, we illustrate this principle through the work of *Hardest Hit*, a community activist coalition in the United Kingdom. We provide practical insights and highlight some of the challenges and lessons learned.

Hardest Hit: Disability activists in London

In 2012, the UK government announced a range of broad austerity measures that included deep cuts to benefits and services for people living with disability and long-term health conditions. Across the United Kingdom, disabled people and their families had already been facing reduced services, a hostile job market and rising costs of everyday living (Cassidy 2012). The announcement galvanised unprecedented community action in what became known as the *Hardest Hit* campaign. Organised jointly by the Disability Benefits Consortium (DBC) and the UK Disabled People's Council, *Hardest Hit* involved a coalition of over 90 organisations and groups of disabled people who came together to fight cuts to disability benefits and protect disabled people's rights and independence.

Hardest Hit strategically mobilised the resources and expertise of its member organisations to produce an extensive report, 'The Tipping Point' (2012) that brought to light shocking new evidence that disabled people are the hardest hit by Government cuts. The report included a survey of over 4,500 disabled people, a poll of more than 350 independent welfare advisors and more than 50 in-depth interviews with disabled people with varying conditions and impairments.

The report was strategically released during the *Hardest Hit*'s highly publicised 2012 'week of action'. Around 100 disabled people joined 100,000 others in a 'march for a better future' through the streets of London, calling on the Government to rethink their cuts to vital services and benefits. Over the following week, *Hardest Hit* events happened throughout the United Kingdom with blind and partially sighted people joining with other disabled people to confront local MPs and policy makers over the cuts.

Community action was organised online through the *Hardest Hit* website, using the online organising tool, e-activist.com, and publicised via the distribution of regular media releases (see Chapter 10). *Hardest Hit* activities and links were publicised on the websites of each member organisation, and via supporters' personal social media pages. Members of *Hardest Hit* also conducted public forums and facilitated smaller-scale community meetings to help organise actions in local communities.

The *Hardest Hit* coalition engaged in sustained action throughout 2013. Involvement of disability organisations and grassroots networks increased. Multiple support groups representing sick and disabled people engaged in online dialogue about the strengths and limitations of proposed policy changes. *Hardest Hit* became recognised by the mass media as valuable source of knowledge and expertise about disability issues. Media coverage about the impacts of government policies on people with disability gradually increased (Hardest Hit Coalition 2013).

The combination of public awareness raising, media coverage, sharing of research evidence and information and direct lobbying of decision-makers helped to raise the profile of disability benefits issues and, importantly, maintain the pressure on parliamentarians to consider modifications to the Welfare Reform Act's cost-cutting measures. By the end of 2013, *Hardest Hit* representatives had developed substantial leverage and were engaged in personal meetings with government ministers (Hardest Hit Coalition 2013). In an important victory for the disability community, *Hardest Hit* had successfully convinced the power-holders that they could not get away with ignoring them.

The story of *Hardest Hit* reminds us that people are most effective in changing the systemic causes of inequity when they engage in collective action. *Hardest Hit* worked by involving small groups, communities, wider networks and professional alliances to mobilise resources and build people's competencies. This large national campaign was made possible through respectful leadership, building partnerships, a strategically planned campaign and by sharing roles and responsibilities amongst community members and experts. The sense of solidarity and mutual support that people gained from this experience also strengthened their confidence about becoming involved with other issues affecting their communities. Regardless of the outcomes, this process has made a substantial contribution to building the capacity of communities and their people for taking an active role in public decision-making in the future.

Collaboration across sectors

The growing focus on social determinants of health and health inequalities opens up a wide range of opportunities for health practitioners and activists to work collaboratively with other sectors and social movements, such as the human rights, environment and labour movements (focused on the rights of workers). By forging strategic connections with other sectors with overlapping interests, health activists are able to strengthen their legitimacy and achieve greater success.

Working on shared agendas provides opportunities to mobilise a larger base of supporters, share knowledge and resources and build on the lessons learned from past success and failures of more established activist groups (Brown et al. 2004). For example, patient support groups have an important role in providing opportunities for people to share information and their experiences of illness and health care. They have also been the crucible for collective action to raise public awareness of the role of complacent governments and irresponsible corporations in contributing to ill-health and injury. Their actions have contributed to closure of the dangerous asbestos industry in many countries and substantial reforms to the safety of workplace conditions for factory and construction workers (Peacock 2009).

Principle 3. Commitment to non-violence

Community activism can change the decisions made by powerful members of government and corporations. At times, this may involve people upholding their right to break the law on the grounds of conscientious objection to something they believe is wrong. For example, occupying a historic site to prevent its destruction or strapping themselves to machinery to prevent its use. While citizens in democracies may want to uphold their right to free speech and public assembly, any action to peacefully break the law should involve a commitment to non-violence and minimal damage to property.

According to Ricketts (2012), this is important for several reasons. First, broad community support is easily alienated through the use of violent or destructive actions. Second, a commitment to non-violent action allows a diverse range of people to participate safely, including the elderly, children and people with disabilities. Third, violent actions will almost always be met with the full violence of the state via police or the military. This can place protestors and community members at risk, undermine the credibility of the cause and reduce the group's likelihood of achieving its goals.

Despite a commitment to non-violence, community members can face consequences, such as arrest, detention, fines and court proceedings, for which they should be well-prepared. This includes being well-informed about the law, police powers and ways of organising protests in order to avoid negative outcomes (Ricketts 2012). For this reason, most community activist groups try to co-opt members with some legal experience into their action group. There are also some excellent guides to organising safe, effective, non-violent action and ways to avoid unnecessary arrests, protect protestors' personal safety and work within their legal rights (see Fitzroy Legal Service 2013; New Tactics in Human Rights 2013; Ricketts 2012).

Violent responses from opponents
It is important to keep in mind that non-violent action, such as a peaceful demonstration, can still result in opponents using injurious force against community members. According to Lakey (2011b), this kind of response is important because can expose the violent nature of power-holders in society. While peaceful protestors do not make the violence happen, their actions raise the underlying injustice to the surface, making visible the violence that was already there in the form of economic inequality and abuses of power and privilege. Media coverage of peaceful protestors being attacked by police or security forces have often been instrumental in shifting public opinion and galvanising widespread public support for community activists and their cause, further strengthening their capacity to bring about social change.

For interested readers, activist and scholar Gene Sharp (2011) provides a fascinating exploration of theory and practice of non-violent action for social change. Another invaluable practical resource is the Global Non-violent Action Database, an online collection with hundreds of case studies of non-violent action (NVA) from almost every country around the world, regularly updated by a team from the Swarthmore University Centre for Peace and Conflict Studies. For more information, go to http://nvdatabase.swarthmore.edu/.

Witness: Video activism, citizen journalism and human rights

Across the world, video activism is a pivotal tool for citizen journalists: that is, community members who use their mobile phones and digital cameras to collect, report and share information about issues of concern. Witness is a New York-based international human rights organization working to build the capacity of citizen journalists to use video in their human rights advocacy campaigns. Established over 20 years ago by musician Peter Gabriel, Witness now provides training and support to local groups in over 80 countries, many of whom live under authoritarian governments and repressive regimes. Their aim is to enable more activists to bring their own stories of human rights abuses into the open, creating videos that become powerful tools for social justice, promoting public engagement and policy change.

Available at no cost to users, the online 'Video for Change Toolkit' contains a range of activist video case studies and takes readers step-by-step through every stage of planning a compelling and effective video to create social change (Witness 2013). Witness has also partnered with the citizen news innovator, Storyful, to create the YouTube Human Rights Channel – a central hub where citizens can upload footage of human rights violations occurring in their communities for the world to see, including those perpetrated against protestors and activists working for social change. For some inspirational insights into the world of human rights video activism, go to www.youtube.com/humanrights.

How activism works in practice

Activism aims to attract public attention, raise awareness about an issue, progressively shift public attitudes and build support for change. By sharing information and networking with others to generate widespread community action, activist groups are able to strengthen their capacity to effectively pressure decision-makers. According to Ricketts (2012), changes to the policy and practices of corporations and governments will be short-lived unless they are grounded in a significant groundswell of community support. Groups of citizens who are well organised are better able to maintain this political pressure in a sustained way until change is achieved. They also have an important watch-dog function to ensure these gains are not reversed over time.

Who are the targets for activism?

The target groups for activist groups are, first, potential members and supporters. This might include people directly affected by the issue, including their family friends and co-workers, but also others concerned about social injustice or what is going 'wrong' in a community or society. Once a critical mass of supporters is achieved, activist groups target those individuals and organisations with the power to influence policies, practices or living and/or working conditions.

As our case studies show, these 'targets' may include high profile individuals, powerful corporations (including their consumers and/or shareholders), governments and local councils, employers and community leaders. In a broader sense, activists also target social norms, embedded practices, policies, or the dominance of certain social groups, such as those who foster patriarchal attitudes towards women, or who tolerate (and even benefit financially from) creating risks to public health (Zoller 2005).

The third target, the media, is a pivotal conduit for contemporary activism. Mass media, alternative media and the Internet facilitate communication between activist groups and their targets. They can also amplify the reach of grass-roots action to a broader audience, helping to mobilise stronger support for the cause. On the other hand, lack of media exposure or unsympathetic media coverage can greatly undermine the effects of any direct action. For this reason, activists need the media knowledge and skills to build and maintain good media relations and to fully utilise the range of available information and communication technologies (ICTs) (Sommerfeldt et al. 2012; Reber & Kim 2006).

Media, public relations and activism

As we noted in chapters 1–4, the contemporary mediasphere is a zone of intense struggle and contestation. Public debates about health and social equity issues are influenced by the priorities and values of not only the decision-makers in organizations and governments, but also the powerful industries and interest groups who seek to influence these decision-makers.

Corporations and governments depend on public relations strategies to manage public perceptions and frame public issues and legislative agendas in ways that advance their interests. Furthermore, whenever their interests are threatened, their public relations departments generate well-orchestrated publicity campaigns in response. Activist groups, therefore, must continually struggle against the well-resourced public relations strategies of their opponents.

Activist groups are inherently at a disadvantage compared to the corporations and governments they seek to influence. They generally have less power, authority, financial resources and access to the mass media for representing their interests to wider society. Consequently, they have unique communication and relationship-building needs (Reber & Kim 2006). Activist groups need to be extremely strategic if they are to influence public opinion and successfully exert pressure on organisations to change problematic policies or practices. Indeed, activist groups are constantly experimenting with developing their own creative PR strategies in order to generate support, discourage opponents' supporters and legitimise their place in the political arena (Derville 2005).

What do activists 'do' and how do they do it?

Strategies and tactics

Activists achieve their goals through a combination of strategies. Some strategies are focused on achieving change whilst others are focused on the survival, growth and sustainability of the group. Tactics are the specific actions and tools used to carry out or implement the strategy.

Strategies and tactics can be grouped as in Table 9.1, although in practice these groupings overlap.

Laverack (2013) explains the range of activist tactics as being a dynamic continuum from indirect, conventional, peaceful actions (such as signing a petition) to more direct and radical tactics.

Activist campaigns are usually carried out in stages, beginning with more conventional indirect actions aimed at awareness-raising and mobilising support. Over time, if it becomes clear that conventional strategies are proving ineffective, groups will progress to more visible direct action to disrupt the target, exert political pressure and/or launch legal action.

The most effective activist organisations use a mix of strategies and tactics to achieve their goals. This approach has several advantages as it

- provides a variety of ways people can get involved according to their interests, abilities and other commitments;
- attracts participation from a greater diversity of community members, including children, the elderly, marginalised groups and people who would not usually consider themselves as 'activists';
- creates more 'newsworthy' opportunities for securing media coverage about the cause; and
- provides multiple points of agitation, disruption and pressure on power-holders that each requires some form of public response (Laverack 2013; Ricketts 2012).

Table 9.1 Activist strategies and tactics

Strategy for raising awareness of the issue and shifting public opinion	Strategy for mobilising support, skills, resources and funding	Strategy for disrupting the target and their usual activities	Strategy for influencing the target by exerting political pressure
Gather and disseminate information. Networking. Generate publicity.	Create opportunities to get involved. Build capacity for action.	Organise visible and/or direct actions.	Pressure decision-makers to change practices, policies or laws.
Tactics and tools	**Tactics and tools**	**Tactics and tools**	**Tactics and tools**
Letters to the editor.	Community liaison with schools, sporting and other community groups.	Consumer boycotts. Peaceful protests.	Petitions and letters to decision-makers. Grassroots lobbying and requests for meetings.
Hold a community meeting. Letter box drops.	Organise tasks and action groups. Workshops to build skills for activism. Fund-raising.	A street march or vigil. Occupy a site, create a blockade.	Media advocacy. Leverage through influential individuals. Direct lobbying of politicians.
Communicate with the public via websites and social media.	Calls for volunteers and donations through social media. Crowd-source funds online.	Picketing, strikes, stopping work and other industrial action. Mass attendance at council meeting. Disrupting a shareholder meeting.	Expose lack of process or conflicts of interest.
Community rallies, music, events and publicity stunts. Establish and build positive media relations			Legal action.

How tactics exert their effect

Indirect actions, such as gathering signatures on a petition, can amount to a significant effect because they demonstrate the strength of public support for change. Direct actions, such as stopworks and boycotts, have a more immediate effect. They can be symbolic and challenging, sending a message to the owners, shareholders and employees of a specific company, and/or to policymakers, about activists' specific concerns (Laverack 2013). This challenge is strengthened if it involves implicit threats of more substantially disruptive action that could undermine the public credibility of an individual or organisation, including public perceptions of their corporate social responsibility. Corporations are especially sensitive to any action that might negatively affect their public image, undermine their profits or result in successful legal action. For this reason, activists try to gather and disseminate information about their opposition that will cause 'reputational damage', thereby forcing them to take more responsible action in order to protect their reputation and ultimately their bottom line (Ricketts 2012).

Opponents' responses to activism

Activism involves communities and ordinary people challenging the authority of more powerful decision-makers and, for this reason, it almost always encounters resistance. For example, employers often oppose workplace reforms because they reduce profits. Worker organisations calling for safer conditions and improved wages have been met with brutal responses from powerful groups whose interests are challenged by activists' struggles for social justice (Qui 2012). Governments and corporations are generally very resilient in the face of public pressure and they are often well-prepared with a suite of tactics to use in response to community activism. As the influence of activist groups on public opinion becomes more powerful, these counter-tactics become increasingly sophisticated.

Examples of counter-tactics include paying experts to speak in the media and launching well-funded advertising campaigns. Governments and corporations also circulate sophisticated media packages to news journalists with material with ready-to-use materials, including press releases, research summaries, comment from experts, audio and video clips (Moynihan & Cassells 2005). Another counter-tactic involves organisations seeking out community groups willing to vouch for their good corporate citizenship and give public credibility to their position against activists. Corporate incentives may be provided in the form of sponsorship of clubs or donations for a new facility, whereas government representatives tend to take a more subtle approach, such as making commitments to address their resource needs via public funding opportunities (Ricketts 2012).

Critical commentators such as Moynihan and Cassels (2005) have provided illuminating research to expose the counter-tactics used by some of the world's biggest companies. This includes establishing their own consumer or patient support groups likely to add legitimacy to their activities (see Chapter 7). Strategies have ranged from providing support for existing 'smokers' rights groups' to the corporate creation of false social media groups with the same intent (Tobacco Tactics 2012). A related tactic called 'astroturfing' is also widely used to create artificial online groups whose members infiltrate social media conversations and defend unpopular corporate activities. Astroturfers actively undermine the opinions and posts of people who challenge their activities (see also Chapter 4).

Corporate tactics to counter activists have even extended to conducting industry-funded health promotion campaigns in order to create an impression of corporate responsibility. For example, multinational tobacco corporation, Philip Morris, funded their own social marketing campaign *Think. Don't Smoke*. The campaign had no success in reducing youth smoking but, not surprisingly, it resulted in more *positive* youth attitudes towards the tobacco industry itself (Farrelly et al. 2002).

Other approaches involve providing financial support for the work of researchers whose findings are likely to support their products, practices or policies. Donations are commonly provided to political parties likely to favour their interests and lawyers are hired to launch legal action against individual members of activist groups (Laverack 2013). It is also common practice for corporations to organise legal challenges to planned policies or existing government regulations (Ricketts 2012).

At the more extreme end of the counter-tactics spectrum, intimidation of individual activists via direct communication, surveillance, harassment and/or threats to their personal safety or property is not uncommon. This tactic has been previously used by some sectors of the pharmaceutical and tobacco industries (Moynihan & Cassells 2005).

In summary, counter-tactics deploy well-resourced public relations strategies to attack the credibility of activist groups and undermine their claims. However, there is good evidence that well-organised and sustained community activism, using multiple strategies and tactics, can have substantial effects (Laverack 2012). Corporations can be pressured to make a commercial decision to withdraw rather than face the reputational damage and growing costs of fighting a public relations battle against communities. Politicians similarly will modify their policy decisions when it becomes clear that the fight is becoming too politically damaging for them (Ricketts 2012). In both cases, activists play an important role in forcing powerful decision-makers to give serious consideration to the community impacts of their policies and practices, as well as the pivotal importance of engaging with communities towards negotiated outcomes.

Working with media

As we note above, the media provide a pivotal conduit for contemporary activism. Mass media, independent media and the Internet facilitate communication between activist groups and various publics. Strategic use of the media helps activist groups to establish their profile and credibility, raise awareness of an issue and present compelling information and evidence. It also enables groups to mobilise a broad base of support, organise collective action and generate publicity to amplify the pressure on decision-makers.

Strategic communication guidelines for activism

Before engaging with the media, health activists need to ensure that all communication is strategically planned to ensure it is accurate, clear and consistent between all spokespersons and across all media, including print, television, radio and online. While each form of communication will need to be tailored for the intended audience, all written materials, in-person interviews and meetings should be guided by a unifying framework.

The following strategic communication guidelines draw on the work of Ricketts (2012) and Reber and Kim (2006).

1. Focus on one issue at a time, rather than multiple aspects of a complex problem.
2. Ensure a positive emphasis explaining how the campaign is advancing the broader public interest, rather than pushing the agenda of a narrow interest group.
3. Carry a clear, simple message:
   o   What is the issue?
   o   Why is it important?
   o   Who are the power-holders? (Which person, organisation or government body has the power to make change possible?)
   o   What outcome is the group seeking?
4. Clearly outline ways people can get involved; ensure that requests for action (often called an 'action alert') are direct and specific.
5. Prepare concise summaries, headings and slogans to reinforce the main message.
6. Utilise a range of media, but always maintain one central website as the control centre and public interface for the organisation and its campaign.
7. Build positive relationships with media professionals, journalists and community media volunteers.
8. Develop a group of media spokespersons for the campaign that includes leaders and community members. A high-profile individual or expert spokesperson can also add considerable leverage. Help them access opportunities to develop media skills such as interviews, speaking in public and fostering good media relations.
9. A practical guide is provided in PHAIWA (2013) and a range of excellent video training materials developed by journalists and public relations professionals are available on YouTube. For an example, go to www. mediafriendly.org.

Mainstream mass media

Mainstream mass media provide opportunities to generate publicity through news, current affairs and feature stories in print, radio, television and online media. They are unrivalled in their ability to reach large audiences and offer great publicity opportunities. However, as we noted in Chapter 4, the intensifying concentration of corporate media ownership has heightened the profit-orientation of most mass media. This increased pressure on journalists to 'produce more with less' has resulted in the vast majority of news stories being sourced directly from public relations materials provided by influential organisations, government bodies and corporate interests. In this context, it is extremely difficult for small organisations to compete. Nonetheless, as we outline below, activist groups can be very creative in developing strong and ongoing relationships with journalists and this can achieve surprisingly good coverage of their campaigns.

Building positive media relations

For activist organisations, a website is instrumental for cultivating good media relations. A website that meets the needs of busy journalists makes it easier for them to cover issues of interest to your organisation. In turn, journalists whose needs are better served by an activist groups' website are more likely to turn to the organisation as an expert source of reliable and easily accessible information when constructing related stories (Sommerfeldt et al. 2012). Characteristics of websites that are most effective in building mutually beneficial relationships between journalists and activist groups include:

- a home page featuring the organisation's mission statement, 'about us' information profiling the organisation and its leaders, the organisation's history and progress to date;
- links to a press room containing resources for journalists, such as press releases, email media kits, searchable archives of media coverage to date, links to recent media stories;
- contact information for experts willing to assist journalists;
- space for journalists to contact the organisation with questions;
- regular email updates circulated to journalists;
- posting of regular news releases and updates;
- links to relevant position papers, background information and publications (Reber & Kim 2006).

Independent media

As we noted in Chapter 4, independent community media provide an important alternative to corporate mass media because they are 'independent' from the influence of profit-oriented media corporations, public relations firms and elite interests. Where mainstream media is driven by commercial imperatives, community media are largely not-for-profit, staffed by volunteers and driven by a public interest focus. Independent media, including community radio and television, tend to be critical and progressive, encouraging activism and attention to social justice issues. These media are generally very willing to carry stories or information about public interest campaigns. They are more likely to provide you with a regular timeslot for community engagement and debate about your campaign, and it is generally easier to mobilise people from an audience-base of citizens already interested in social action (Howley 2010). For readers interested in finding out more about independent community media, Chapter 7 takes a more in-depth look at their importance for health promotion and provides practical insights into the ways these media are used by ethnic communities, indigenous groups, prisoners, LGBTI communities and people living with disabilities.

Generating your own media

There are numerous possibilities for activist groups to generate their own media using Internet and digital technologies in order to build support and generate community action. Even for small community action groups, a website is essential as the central coordination hub and also for providing the public interface for the organisation and its campaign. A number of activism host organisations provide an online portal and step-by-step frameworks to help groups set up a campaign website and plan their campaigns. Examples can be found at www.causes.com and www.change.org. Some host organisations also provide options to help groups use crowd-sourcing as a way of generating donations from the public to support their work. Some of the most established not-for-profit crowd-funding sites include indiegogo.com and fundrazr.com.

At a more local level, other common approaches used by activist groups to generate their own media include organising a regular spot on a community radio or TV station (see chapters 6 and 7). It is also useful to produce a short video that contains key messages and images for distribution via Facebook and YouTube. Community members can be invited to create their own campaign video and a selection of these may be posted on the main campaign website. All digital outputs can be cross-linked so they can be easily shared by anyone who views them on Twitter, Facebook or YouTube. Many groups build an email list and informal SMS network through which to publicise and communicate (Ricketts 2012).

Online activism using social media, mobile and digital technologies also contributes significantly to increasing the reach and effectiveness of activist campaigns, providing an inexpensive way to engage large numbers of people who may not otherwise be concerned about the issue (Shaw 2013). Within a very short timeframe, mass action to pressure decision-makers can be facilitated through online petitions, Twitter protests and circulation of action alerts (calls for action) that achieve exponential responses through links with other social media pages. To see how this works in practice, go to www.greenpeace.org and the examples in Hefler et al. (2013) and PHAIWA (2013).

As we noted in Chapter 4, interactive digital media create a wide range of opportunities for enhancing existing linkages between people and communities, not only to share knowledge and resources, but also to strengthen support between people trying to create positive social change. Opportunities are created for engaging communities in problem-solving by creating new networks and also by weaving together existing networks of groups not normally accustomed to working together to create new sources of inspiration and power to address health and social issues. For example, video generated by activist groups and their supporters has had an increasingly important security role in public rallies, demonstrations and direct action. Mobile phones and sophisticated monitoring technologies are frequently used to ensure that any violence and human rights abuses against protestors are well-documented (Andrejevic 2011).

Recent research by Hefler and colleagues (2013) provides insights for online activism using social media platforms such as Facebook, Twitter and Change. Their research also demonstrated that effective youth activism depends on having opportunities for public dialogue; social media platforms moderated by a representative from the group can provide valuable opportunities for robust debate about the campaign approach, offering a chance for activist groups to engage with its critics and argue in defence of their campaigns. Several useful practical guides to online activism can also be found in Shaw (2013), Ricketts (2012) and online at www.thechangeagency.org and www.newtactics.org.

Practical planning

Strategy: The key to effective activism

Strategic planning is the key to effective activism. Passionate, energetic and committed groups of people can often generate a great deal of interest and community action, but people often confuse a successful tactic with a successful outcome. Activist groups are unlikely to have an impact on decision-makers unless the campaign has been carefully mapped out and all elements coordinated to achieve success.

Ricketts (2012) recommends using an integrated strategy map to help all participants stay focused on the big picture (goal and objectives) and understand how activities at every stage (tactics) fit into that picture. Following Ricketts' (2012: 52) framework, we provide an example integrated strategy plan in Figure 9.1. This diagram illustrates the approach taken by the campaign *Burger Off! No McDonalds in the Dandenong Ranges*, developed by a small Australian community fighting to keep the giant multinational, McDonald's corporation, out of their town (Burger Off 2014). For more details about the specific tactics and tools used in this inspirational campaign, go to www. burgeroff.org (Figure 9.1).

Starting up or 'revitalising' an activism campaign

Most activist campaigns start from small beginnings, often one or two concerned individuals who start a conversation, spread the word, gather people together and gradually develop a plan of action. Based on years of experience working with local activist groups, Ricketts (2012) suggests the following ten questions to help guide these early, formative stages of campaign planning. They begin with a set of intuitive questions useful for brainstorming, and each leads to more concrete decision-making that will help to develop a more formal, integrated campaign strategy (Table 9.2).

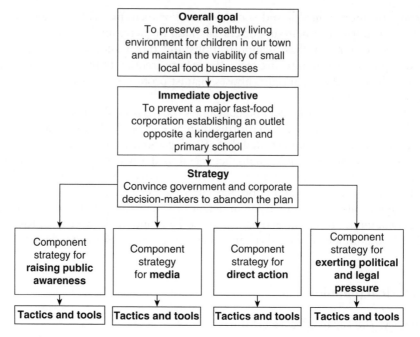

Figure 9.1   Integrated strategy plan example

Source: Adapted from Ricketts (2012: 52)

Table 9.2   Campaign planning: Ten key questions

Intuitive question	Strategic consideration
1. What is the issue/problem?	What is our overall goal and immediate objective(s)?
2. What do we want to do about it?	What strategies will we use?
3. How will we achieve this?	What tactics can we use?
4. Who will do what?	Allocate tasks and responsibilities
5. Whom do we need to convince?	Who are the relevant power-holders?
6. What more do we need to know?	What further research do we need to do (or locate)?
7. What skills and resources are available?	What resources do we have (or need to obtain)?
8. Who can help us?	Whom can we form alliances with or seek assistance from?
9. How much time do we have?	What timelines should we set?
10. What could go wrong?	How do we plan for the unexpected?

Source: Adapted from Ricketts (2012: 60)

Practical tips for effective activism

Drawing on the contents of this chapter, and its underpinning literature, a summary of practical tips for effective activism at each of the key stages is provided as follows.

Getting started
Develop a small working group. Build trust and cooperation by deciding on leadership and basic protocols about how the group will function (see Ricketts 2012). Focus on raising awareness and recruiting other interested participants. To help the group become more organised, consider utilising the interests of various members by forming smaller action groups with specific roles. Aim to build the skills and confidence of participants. Focus on engaging community partners and involving external allies and elites (Laverack 2013).

Planning the campaign
Follow the process outlined above to help the group set goals and objectives. Identify 'powerholders' who are likely to be opponents of the campaign and also those likely to be supporters (see Chapter 10; see also Ricketts 2012). The next step is to select the mix of strategies and tactics to help achieve these objectives. This will, in part, be guided by the resources and time available but should also be informed by available evidence about what has been effective in other related campaigns (Laverack 2013; Freudenberg et al. 2009). Focus on setting timelines and mobilising resources.

Communicating the message
Continue to research the issue and gather further evidence to support the campaign objectives and strategies. Develop information and a range of communication materials for various public audiences and specific decision-makers. Ensure these are regularly reviewed and updated (PHAIWA 2013; Ricketts 2012). Focus on building positive media relations and generating publicity (Chapman 2007; see also Chapter 10). Aim to build the group's capacity for political pressure by linking up with existing networks, alliances and coalitions. Consider ways to involve influential people with leverage and/or lobbying skills (Laverack 2013; see also Chapter 10).

Monitoring, evaluation and sustainability
In order to keep up the fight, the group should plan strategies for survival, growth and sustainability. Ongoing monitoring and evaluation are essential. Ensure the group's activities (process and outcomes) are carefully recorded, monitored and evaluated. As we have discussed earlier in this chapter, a central principle of activism is the empowerment of people and communities. Regardless of the final campaign outcomes, it is crucially important to evaluate participants' perspectives about the process of empowerment and building community capacity to collectively identify and address issues of concern. Freudenberg et al. (2011) provide an excellent guide for practitioners in this regard.

It is important to document every success, no matter how small and ensure these are widely publicised. Keep records of people involved, media coverage, tactics used and opponents' responses (see PHAIWA 2013). Work towards fostering positive, ongoing media relations and maintain a strong online presence for the group, its activities and potential supporters (Shaw 2013; Ricketts 2012). All contact with media and coverage should be recorded (date, media type, publication name, author, headline, spokesperson, subject and/or news angle). Media coverage should be archived and links made available on the campaign website (Chapman 2007; Reber & Kim 2006). Be creative about ways to locate resources and funding independent of government or corporate vested interests. And finally, be persistent: effective activism requires a range of strategies by a variety of groups and organisations over a sustained period of time.

What role do health practitioners have in activism?

To close this chapter, we reflect on the range of potential roles for health practitioners in activism and community action as leaders, supporters, facilitators and expert mediators. Practitioners have an important role as facilitators, helping people to access the resources, knowledge and skills they need to organise effective activism campaigns. Health promotion practitioners' expertise in accessing sound evidence to support the key arguments presented in activist groups' campaign can provide invaluable resource for effectively communicating a clear and powerful message to the public, the media and their 'targets'. Health practitioners often have a role in helping people to gain more understanding of policy-making and how they can how they can influence this process. Health practitioners' understanding of activism principles and practice can help community groups to decide whether activism is an appropriate strategy, understand its strengths and limitations and take steps for getting started.

In some cases, health practitioners cannot be directly involved in activism, particularly if the issue is controversial or involves lobbying their own organisation (Gould et al. 2012). Nevertheless, they can provide support for activists by locating evidence to support the proposed solution, helping to interpret this evidence and making key findings more understandable for the general public. Practitioners also assist activist groups by advising them about government health priorities, policies and recently released reports that provide support for their changes they are seeking. Their affiliations with various professional associations, local health services and educational organisations provide valuable opportunities to help activist groups access resources for conducting community forums and training sessions.

Health practitioners also have an important mediating role between (less powerful) community activist groups and those (more powerful) groups with decision-making authority in local councils, health organisations, governments and a range of industries that affect health. For groups, or issues, that might otherwise be dismissed by decision-makers as being unimportant, health practitioners can add a level of expertise that lends legitimacy to the cause on health grounds. Their professional links with health-related networks and coalitions can assist groups to collaborate with other sectors with shared interests or overlapping agendas, such as food industries and parents' groups concerned about childhood obesity. In summary, while there have been a number of remarkable health professional activist leaders, the most important role of health professionals is not to take over leadership of a community group, but to be a supporter and facilitator, helping to empower communities and their people so they can actively participate in driving their own agenda for social change and health improvement.

CHAPTER SUMMARY

- Health activism aims to achieve changes in the policies and practices of governments, corporations and other organisations. It works by getting issues onto the public agenda and generating community action to put pressure on decision-makers whose policies or practices affect them adversely.

- Health activism can be distinguished from other forms of public health advocacy because it is commonly conducted outside formal institutionalised political channels.

- There is good evidence that well-organised and sustained community activism, using multiple strategies and tactics, can have substantial effects.

- Health activism is underpinned by the idea that educated, empowered and organised groups of citizens have an important role in creating healthy social change. Key principles include empowerment and participation; collective action through community organising; and a commitment to non-violence.

- Health activism works to address social injustice through engaging and empowering communities and their people so they can actively participate in driving their own agenda for social change and health improvement. Activism can also be a mechanism for addressing inequity and building stronger communities through increasing community participation and influence on decision-making.

- Governments and corporations are generally very resilient in the face of public pressure, and they are often well prepared with a suite of tactics to use in response to community activism.

- Activist groups are inherently at a disadvantage compared to the corporations and governments they seek to influence. Consequently, they need to be extremely strategic if they are to influence public opinion and successfully exert pressure on organisations to change problematic policies or practices.

- The media is a pivotal conduit for contemporary activism. Mass media, alternative media and the Internet facilitate communication between activist groups and their targets. They can also amplify the reach of grass-roots action to a broader audience, helping to mobilise stronger support for the cause. Activists need the media knowledge and skills to build and maintain good media relations and to fully utilise the range of available information and communication technologies.

References

Al Jazeera 2013, 'Saudi prince makes case for women drivers', 15 April. Accessed 6 May 2014 http://www.aljazeera.com/news/middleeast/2013/04/201341415473271705.html.

Anderson, H. 2012, Facilitating active citizenship: Participating in prisoners' radio. *Critical Studies in Media Communication*, 1–15. doi:10.1080/15295036.2012.688212.

Andrejevic, M. 2011, 'Watching back: Surveillance as activism', in S. Curry Jansen, J. Pooley and L. Taub-Pervizpour (eds), *Media and Social Justice*, Palgrave Macmillan, New York.

Brown, P. and Zavestoski, S. 2004, 'Social movements in health: An introduction', *Socioloogy of Health and Illness*, 26 (6): 679–694.

Brown, P., Zavestoski, S., McCormick, S., Mayer, B., Morello-Frosch, R. and Altman, R. 2004, 'Embodied health movements: New approaches to social movements in health', *Sociology of Health and Illness*, 26 (1): 50–80.

Burger Off 2014, www.burgeroff.org.

Cassidy, S. 2012, 'More than 300,000 disabled people to have benefits cut says Esther McVey', *The Independent*, 13 December. Accessed 6 May 2014 http://www.independent.co.uk/news/uk/politics/more-than-300000-disabled-people-to-have-benefits-cut-says-esther-mcvey-8413498.html.

Chapman, S. 2007, *Public Health Advocacy and Tobacco Control: Making Smoking History*, Blackwell, Oxford.

Crossier, S. 2012, 'John Snow: The London cholera epidemic of 1854', *Center for Spatially integrated Social Science*. Accessed 6 May 2014 www.csiss.org/classics.

Curry Jansen, S., Pooley, J. and Taub-Pervizpour, L. 2011, *Media and Social Justice*, Palgrave Macmillan, New York.

Derville, T. 2005, 'Radical activist tactics: Overturning public relations conceptualizations', *Public Relations Review*, 31: 527–533.

Dutta, M. J. 2011, *Communicating Social Change: Structure, Culture, and Agency*, Routledge, New York.

English, F. W. 2007, 'Alinsky, Saul (1909–1972)', in G. L. Andersen and K. G. Herr (eds), *Encyclopedia of Activism and Social Justice*, Sage Publications, London.

Every Australian Counts 2013. Accessed 6 May 2014 www.everyaustraliancounts.com.au.

Farrelly, M., Healton, C., Davis, K., Messeri, P., Hersey, J. and Haviland, L. 2002, 'Getting to the truth: Evaluating National Tobacco Countermarketing Campaigns', *American Journal of Public Health*, 92 (6): 901–907.

Fitzroy Legal Service 2013. Accessed 6 May 2014 www.activistsrights.org.au.

Freudenberg, N., Bradley, S. and Serrano, M. 2009, 'Public health campaigns to change industry practices that damage health: An analysis of 12 case studies', *Health Education and Behaviour*, 36 (2): 230–249.

Freudenberg, N., Pastor, M. and Israel, B. 2011, 'Strengthening community capacity to participate in making decisions to reduce disproportionate environmental exposures', *American Journal of Public Health*, 101 (1): 123–130.

Gould, T., Fleming, M. and Parker, E. 2012, 'Advocacy for health: Revisiting the role of health promotion', *Health Promotion Journal of Australia*, 23 (3): 165–170.

Hardest Hit 2012, 'The tipping point: The human and economic costs of cutting disabled people's support'. Accessed 6 May 2014 http://www.rnib.org.uk/getinvolved/campaign/yourmoney/Documents/HH_TippingPoint.pdf .

Hardest Hit Coalition 2013, 'Hardest hit: Our rights, our independence, our lives'. Accessed 6 May 2014 http://thehardesthit.wordpress.com/about.

Hefler, M., Freeman, B. and Chapman, S. 2013, 'Tobacco control advocacy in the age of social media: Using Facebook, Twitter and Change', *Tobacco Control*, 22 (3): 210–214.

Holland, K., Blood, W., Pirkis, J. and Dare, A. 2009, 'Postpsychiatry in the Australian media: The 'vulnerable' talk back', *Asia Pacific Media Educator*, June 2008/July 2009, (19): 143–157.

Howley, K. 2010, *Understanding Community Media*, Sage, Los Angeles.

Human Rights Watch 2013, World Report 2013: Saudi Arabia. Accessed 6 May 2014 http://www.hrw.org/world-report/2013/country-chapters/saudi-arabia.

Keleher, H. 2011, 'Health education for empowerment', in H. Keleher and C. MacDougall (eds), *Understanding Health*, 3rd Edition, Oxford, Melbourne, 235–247.

Lakey, G. 2011a, 'Non-violent action defined', *Global Non-Violent Action Database*, http://nvdatabase.swarthmore.edu/content/non-violent action defined.

Lakey, G. 2011b, 'Issue clusters', *Global Non-Violent Action Database*, http://nvdatabase.swarthmore.edu/issue-clusters.

Laverack, G. 2012, 'Health activism', *Health Promotion International*, 27 (4): 429–434.

Laverack, G. 2013, *Health Activism: Foundations and Strategies*, Sage, London.

Lewis, J. 2008, *Cultural Studies,* 2nd Edition, Sage, London.

Lewis, J. and Lewis, B. 2009, *Bali's Silent Crisis: Desire, Tragedy and Transition*, Lexington Books, Rowman and Littlefield, Lanham, MD.

Liu, N. 2011, 'Colombians use sex strike to get highway repaired', *Global Non-violent Action Database*, www.nvdatabase.swarthmore.edu/content/colombians-use-sex-strike-get-highway-repaired-huelga-de-piernas-cruzada-2011.

Marmot Review 2010, 'Fair society, healthy lives: Strategic review of health inequalities in England Post-2010', *Executive Summary*. Accessed 6 May 2014 www.marmotreview.org.

Minkler, M. and Wallerstein, N. (eds) 2010, *Community-Based Participatory Research for Health: From Process to Outcomes*, Wiley, San Francisco.

Moynihan, R. and Cassells, A. 2005, *Selling Sickness: How the World's Biggest Drug Companies Are Turning Us All into Patients*, Allen & Unwin, Crows Nest.

Nathanson, C. and Hopper, K. 2010, 'The Marmot review – Social revolution by stealth', *Social Science and Medicine*, 71 (7): 1237–1239.

New Tactics in Human Rights 2013, www.newtactics.org.

Peacock, M. 2009, *Killer Company*, ABC Books, Melbourne.

Pollitt, K. 2013, 'Saudi Human Rights Activist Wajeha Al-Huwaider sentenced to Prison', *The Nation*, 19 June. Accessed 6 May 2014 http://www.thenation.com/blog/174894/saudi-human-rights-activist-wajeha-al-huwaider-sent-prison#.

Public Health Advocacy Institute of Western Australia 2013, *Public Health Advocacy Toolkit*, 3rd Edition, Curtin University, Perth. Accessed 6 May 2014 www.phaiwa.org.au.

Qui, J. 2012, 'Network labour: Beyond the shadow of Foxconn', in L. Hjorth, J. Burgess and I. Richardson (eds), *Studying Mobile Media Cultural Technologies, Mobile Communication, and the iPhone*, Routledge, New York, 173–189.

Reber, B. and Kim, J. 2006, 'How activist groups use websites in media relations: Evaluating online press rooms', *Journal of Public Relations Research*, 18 (2): 313–333.

Ricketts, A. 2012, *The Activists Handbook: A Step-By-Step Guide to Participatory Democracy*, Zed Books, London.

Sharp, G. 2011, *Sharp's Dictionary of Power and Struggle*, Oxford University Press, United Kingdom.

Shaw, R. 2013, The *Activist's Handbook: Winning Social Change in the 21st Century*, 2nd Edition, University of California Press, Berkeley.

Snow, S. 1999, 'Death by Water: John Snow and Cholera in the Nineteenth Century', *Liverpool Medical Institution*, http://www.lmi.org.uk/Data/10/Docs/11/11Snow.pdf.

Sommerfeldt, E., Kent, M. and Taylor, M. 2012, 'Activist practitioner perspectives of *website* public relations: Why aren't activist websites fulfilling the dialogic promise?', *Public Relations Review*, 38 (2): 303–312.

The Change Agency n.d., http://www.thechangeagency.org.

Tobacco Tactics 2012, 'Astroturfing', *Tobacco Tactics*. Accessed 6 May 2014 http://tobaccotactics.org/index.php?title=Astroturfing.

Toumi, H. 2013, 'Saudi woman disguises as man to drive bus', *Gulf News*, 25 February, http://gulfnews.com/news/gulf/saudi-arabia/saudi-woman-disguises-as-man-to-drive-bus-1.1150721.

Video Volunteers 2013. Accessed 6 May 2014 http://www.videovolunteers.org.

WHO 1978, 'Declaration of Alma-Ata'. Accessed 6 May 2014 http://www.who.int/publications/almaata_declaration_en.pdf

WHO 1986, Ottawa charter for health promotion, in WHO 2009, *Milestones in Health Promotion: Statements from Global Conferences*, WHO/NMH/CHP/09.01, 1–5. Accessed 6 May 2014 http://www.who.int/healthpromotion/Milestones_Health_Promotion_05022010.pdf.

WHO 1998, 'Health Promotion Glossary', *World Health Organization*, Geneva, www.who.int/hpr.

WHO 2008, *The World Health Report 2008: Primary Health Care – Now More than Ever*, World Health Organization, Geneva.

Wilkinson, R. and Pickett, K. 2010, *The Spirit Level: Why Equality Is Better for Everyone*, 2nd Edition, Penguin Books, London.

Witness 2013, 'Video for Change Toolkit', http://www.witness.org/how-to.

Zoller, H. M. 2005, 'Health activism: Communication theory and action for social change', *Communication Theory*, 15 (4): 341–364.

Advocacy for Healthy Public Policy

10

Chapter overview

In this chapter, we introduce the principles and practice of public health advocacy using a range of practical examples. We draw on the real-life experiences of practitioners to illustrate some of the challenges and lessons learned from their often extraordinarily tenacious efforts to influence government policy and corporate practices. The chapter outlines simple frameworks for advocacy planning and describes a range of strategies and practical tools for more effective public health advocacy. This chapter builds on the content of the Chapter 9 ('Health Activism'). Both are designed as companion chapters. Advocacy and activism share similar goals, but they adopt different approaches. They are like two sides of the same coin: mutually complementary strategies that depend on one another to work synergistically. For this reason, we recommend readers begin with Chapter 9 before progressing to this chapter.

Introduction

Advocacy has a pivotal role in advancing population health by influencing decision-makers who have the power to create healthy public policy. The goal of public health advocacy is to create social, physical and legislative environments that make it easier for people to be healthy (Gould et al. 2012). Advocacy involves practitioners and community members working together for change. We begin this chapter with a recent case study. It tells the story of a passionately committed alliance between workers, patient groups, health practitioners and human rights advocates and their efforts to force government action over the deadly asbestos industry.

A deadly workplace: Asbestos victims fight for social justice

Asbestos is a fibrous material that was widely used building construction after the Second World War. Since that time, thousands of workers have contracted asbestosis, cancers and other life-threatening illnesses caused by exposure to the product. Patient support groups have worked with unionists and lawyers to successfully launch legal action for compensation from asbestos producers after revelations that company executives had been well aware of the dangers, but had concealed this knowledge for decades (Peacock 2009). Along with their families and supporters, men affected by disease have also worked in an advocacy role with the environmental and occupational justice movements to push for complete bans on the asbestos industry in the United Kingdom, the United States, Canada and Australia.

In 2011, the Canadian government was still approving the production and sale of asbestos to India for widespread use in poor communities for housing construction. Concerned advocates called upon their established networks and alliances to launch action to push for change. In India, where the use of asbestos is still legal, activists and health workers ran workshops across the country to gather local 'lay' evidence from many hundreds of workers and community members about negative health effects. They also photographed children playing in deadly tailings dams and inhaling contaminated dust (Peacock 2011).

With the support of several committed journalists, this story attracted extensive media attention, raising public awareness about the Canadian government's failure to stop the highly profitable transfer of health risks to some of the world's most disadvantaged people. With an election in the same year, widespread public condemnation helped to intensify political pressure. It also added weight to the advocacy coalition's threat of launching legal action based on human rights grounds. In September 2012, Pauline Marois, the newly elected premier in the Province of Quebec, Canada, fulfilled her election promise to finally put a complete halt to the mining and export of asbestos (Chappell 2012).

The above example illustrates how alliances between patient groups, health practitioners and the environment and labour movements can add significant leverage to their fight for social justice. This campaign generated public support through extensive media coverage and lobbied decision-makers with a combination of expert evidence and lay epidemiology. Effectiveness of the campaign was strengthened by building on the success of previous legal action. Timing of the campaign was strategically planned for the months leading up to an important election in order to ensure it had maximum political impact.

By incorporating a sound understanding of the theory, key principles and practical frameworks that underpin effective advocacy, health practitioners played an important role in the success of this campaign. As Gould et al. (2012) have noted, many health practitioners appreciate the importance of advocacy but lack the confidence and skills to incorporate it into their work. Accordingly, the next section will explore the fundamentals of public health advocacy and the communication strategies needed to apply these principles in practice.

Understanding public health advocacy

What is public health advocacy?

Public health advocacy is a process of gaining political commitment for change. More specifically, it aims to achieve policy changes to support initiatives that address the underlying causes of ill-health and inequalities in health. Advocacy uses strategic communication to shape debates, shift public opinion, exert political pressure and influence the decision-makers with responsibility for laws, regulations or policies that affect health (Gould et al. 2012).

In the previous chapter, we explored *activism*, a strategy that aims to raise critical consciousness amongst community members and generate widespread grass-roots action to pressure decision-makers. *Advocacy* is the more formal part of the process. It aims to ensure the work of activists is effectively translated into changes in government policies and corporate practices.

In contrast to health *activism*, which commonly involves community groups operating outside institutionalised channels of political influence, public health *advocacy* works within the system by strategically using the media, political lobbying and mobilising coalitions and alliances.

Advocacy is a form of communication that involves 'taking a position on an issue, and initiating actions in a deliberate attempt to influence private and public policy choices' (Labonte 1994 in Gould 2012). Health advocacy has been defined as actions intended to achieve 'political commitment, policy support, social acceptance and systems support for a particular health goal or programme' (World Health Organization 1998). Both of these definitions emphasise the importance of health practitioners becoming actively engaged in political processes to bring about change. These definitions are underpinned by the notion that 'improving public health requires an *explicit commitment* to advocating for policy changes that support the development of health promoting environments' (Johnson 2009: 1). Put simply, public health advocacy is 'a strategy for blending science and politics with a social justice value orientation to make the system work better, particularly for those with the least resources' (Wallack et al. 1999: 7).

Advocacy success stories: What can public health advocacy achieve?

According to Chapman (2007: 1226), 'every branch of public health can point to the critical role of advocacy in translating research into policy practice and sea changes in public opinion'. The targets for public health advocacy include (Chapman 1994: 6):

• policies and practices of governments and institutions whose actions affect the lives of many people;
• laws and government regulations;

- the commercial marketing practices of industries; and
- the activities of counter-health lobby groups who, if successful in their aims, can delay or obstruct initiatives to improve public health.

Public health advocacy campaigns have been pivotal in bringing about advances in healthy public policy. Notable examples include mandatory removal of lead from petrol; more consistent labelling of additives and nutritional content of food products; innovative taxation policies to support health promotion initiatives; and injury prevention policies such as compulsory seat-belts in cars (Chapman 1994). Groundbreaking gun law reforms in Australia have led to a 59.9% decrease in male gun-related suicides and the complete absence of mass shootings during the 17 years since their introduction (Chapman 2013). In United Kingdom, Australia, parts of Europe and the United States, advocates for stronger tobacco control policy have been a powerful driving force behind the successful introduction of bans on tobacco advertising and promotion, mass-reach public awareness campaigns, taxes on tobacco products to reduce demand and controls on smoking in public places. Sustained tobacco control advocacy over several decades has achieved the policy changes necessary for substantial reductions in smoking levels to almost 20% in a number of countries (Chapman 2007).

Public health researchers and practitioners have also used advocacy as a catalyst for government action to address broader issues of social inequity. This has been achieved by (i) focusing public attention towards the social determinants of health problems and (ii) advocating for policies to support disadvantaged communities through improved access to education, fair work opportunities, safe housing, affordable healthy foods and public transport (see Laverack 2013).

At the community level, health practitioners have used advocacy to become involved in local government decision-making about policies that affect health. Groups of concerned doctors have successfully lobbied for regulations to make swimming pool fences compulsory (Orlowski 1989), nutritionists have helped parent groups advocate for healthier menus in school canteens (Parents Jury 2013); and occupational therapists have won hard-fought battles for policy to stop young people with brain injuries being forced to live in aged care homes (Summer Foundation 2013).

Why advocacy is essential in the fight for public health

The role of advocacy
Public health advocacy can be extremely contentious because it occurs at the intersection of major social, political, economic and cultural forces in society (Johnson 2009). Many public health policy interventions involve changing laws, regulations, policies, taxes, prices and product standards, so it is inevitable that they are rarely implemented without challenge. Public health initiatives are often opposed by various elements of government, industry and even other health sectors concerned about shifting the allocation of scarce

public resources or imposing policies and regulations that could potentially work against their interests.

Most major public health policy and legislative initiatives have only been successfully implemented after extended periods of news coverage, public discussion and political debate (Chapman 2007). Within this context, public health advocates must compete for prominence in a highly contested political arena – often in the face of highly organised opposition (Chapman 2004).

The central role of the media

As we noted in the first four chapters of this book, the media has a central social, cultural and political role in society, and it is also a pivotal conduit for contemporary political processes. Through the media, well-resourced politicians and vested interest groups deploy sophisticated public relations activities to build favourable public opinion for their political positions and preferred policies. This means that advocates for public health initiatives also need to make strategic use of the media to influence news coverage, public discussion and political debate between supporters and opponents (Chapman 2007).

As we noted in Chapter 9, mass media, community media and social media all have an important role in facilitating communication between advocates and the decision-makers they are seeking to influence. They also help to amplify the reach of advocacy efforts to a broader audience, helping to mobilise stronger public support for change. However, lack of media exposure or unsympathetic media coverage can greatly undermine the effects of any advocacy campaign. For this reason, public health practitioners and researchers need the media knowledge and skills to strategically use various media to achieve their advocacy goals.

How does advocacy fit into existing frameworks for health promotion?

The World Health Organization endorses the pivotal importance of advocacy in health promotion: 'Progress toward a healthier world requires strong political action, broad participation and sustained advocacy' (WHO 2005). Gould et al. (2012: 165) reiterate the WHO position that 'health professionals have a major responsibility to act as advocates for health at all levels in society' and 'health systems have the power and duty to advocate for healthy public policies across government and address the structural determinants of health'. Whether health practitioners are seeking to influence decisions made in small local councils or at much higher levels of government, advocacy skills are critical to effective health promotion practice.

Public health advocacy is considered to be an upstream approach to communicating for health promotion. Rather than a focus on changing individual knowledge, attitudes and behaviour, it seeks to change the broader context for people's health choices by influencing the social, economic, legislative environments in which individual choices take place (Chapman 1994). Its primary objective is to shift the focus of decision-makers from traditional individualistic, victim-blaming and medicalised approaches to health problems towards

Table 10.1 Difference between advocacy and social marketing campaigns

Advocacy	Social marketing
Mobilises community activists and influences decision-makers	Motivates/persuades people to undertake personal change
Emphasis on social responsibility	Emphasis on individual responsibility
Influence on environments through policy changes	Influence on individual behaviour
Uses news media, political lobbying and coalitions for action.	Uses information and education, persuasive marketing and paid advertising

more upstream public health approaches that address disadvantage and create healthier environments for everyone.

Green and Tones (2010) illustrate this 'shift' by contrasting two approaches to tackling inequalities in health associated with smoking. One approach is to provide education and specifically targeted health messages to reach disadvantaged groups. The other uses advocacy to 'challenge the social and political system that results in disadvantage in the first place' (p.389). Table 10.1 illustrates some of the differences between advocacy and traditional social marketing approaches to using the media in public health (Table 10.1).

Skills and competencies for advocacy
Effective public health advocacy requires a combination of skills and competencies. According to Gould et al. (2012), these include:

- understanding policy and programme decision-making processes (how policy decisions are made and who makes them);
- developing evidence-based and persuasive arguments for change;
- communicating effectively with government and political officials;
- working with the media to frame issues, present solutions and generate public support;
- working with alliances and coalitions of stakeholder groups to leverage further political pressure; and
- empowering community members to participate in advocacy and local decision-making.

We illustrate the importance of these skills below by profiling a recent advocacy campaign in which health professionals, health promotion practitioners and community action groups worked together to change the practices of a powerful and high-profile corporation.

Challenging unhealthy advertising tactics: Small coalition versus a corporate giant
In 2008, three public health advocacy groups in Australia – the Obesity Policy Coalition, the Parents Jury consumer group and the Australian Dental Association – launched an advocacy campaign to challenge the giant multinational corporation, Coca-Cola. They worked together to lodge a formal complaint to the Australian government's Competition and Consumer Commission (ACCC)

over Coca-Cola's advertising campaign targeting mothers and children. The ads featured a well-known actress and mother, Kerry Armstrong, who adopted a myth-busting role to dismiss concerns about the product being unhealthy. Common 'myths' were listed: Coke 'makes you fat', 'rots your teeth' and 'is packed with caffeine'. The ads then provided the company's version of the 'facts' to counter these apparent misunderstandings by the general public. Several months later, in early 2009, the ACCC issued a court-enforceable order against Coca-Cola forcing them to withdraw the ads and publish a series of corrective advertisements. Each advocacy group issued media releases to draw journalist's attention to the issue and secure media coverage in order to publicise their success. Considerable media coverage was generated and this created further opportunities to promote public health initiatives to address the underlying causes of obesity. By working with government regulatory agencies and the media, the campaign was able to expose the company's misleading marketing practices; reinforce health messages about links between soft drink consumption, weight gain and tooth decay; and add momentum to the campaign for improved food-labelling standards and stronger regulation of the advertising industry (Public Health Advocacy Institute of Western Australia (PHAIWA) 2013b). More information can be obtained from the Obesity Policy Coalition at www.opc.org.au.

Principles of public health advocacy

As the above case studies illustrate, effective public health advocacy campaigns share common characteristics. Several key principles for public health advocacy are outlined briefly as follows:

1. Expect opposition
Advocacy is almost always contested by opponents of change. Advocates should get to know who their opponents are, their position on the issue and their key arguments, then devise strategies for countering them. Well-resourced and powerful opponents can be challenged by harnessing the power of public authorities, regulatory bodies and government commissions of enquiry, particularly those with the capacity to enforce laws and/or undertake legal action (Ricketts 2012; Freudenberg et al. 2009; Chapman 2007).

2. Recognise different perspectives
Stakeholder groups have various different perspectives on the problem advocates are seeking to address and the solutions they are proposing. The role of advocacy is to 'frame' problems and solutions in ways that identify social and environmental causes, attribute responsibility and generate support for healthy public policy (Freudenberg et al. 2009; Wallack et al. 1999).

3. Look for opportunities
Advocates need to be creative, controversial and at times unpopular, if they are to be vanguards of change (Chapman 2007). Advocacy can be 'proactive' or 'reactive'. Working proactively often involves bringing issues onto the public

agenda, including unrecognised public health issues or those being strategically overlooked by decision-makers. Reactive advocacy, on the other hand, responds to things that happen. It looks for windows of opportunity that might provide the catalyst for change. This can involve responding to media news, entertainment or advertising content (PHAIWA 2013a). Even a serious event, personal tragedy or disaster provides an opportunity to present arguments about upstream causes and how policy change could prevent these in the future. As Chapman (2013) argues in his powerful book about Australia's fight for gun law reforms, a mass shooting or the accidental death of a child is an undeniable tragedy, but horrors such as these have also provided the catalyst for advocates to successfully galvanise public opinion and political commitment for change. Committed advocates have a responsibility to be alert to crisis, prepared in advance and ready to respond.

4. Be strategic, purposeful and persistent

Effective advocacy involves sustained action, long timeframes, multiple strategies and well-organised coalitions and alliances. The most successful campaigns are strategically planned with clear objectives but also flexible enough to respond to unfolding events. Timing is paramount and advocates often start campaigning many months before elections, deadlines for public submissions on important policy issues and release dates for budgets and major reports. Successful policy change is most often achieved through a series of small wins, so advocacy groups need to be unrelentingly persistent (Freudenberg et al. 2009; Chapman 2007).

5. Accuracy and evidence are paramount

Governments, politicians and the public are influenced by credible organisations who present powerful, evidence-based arguments for change that are communicated in ways they can understand. All facts and figures used in public statements or written information should be simple, accurate and backed up by expert opinion and high-quality, peer-reviewed sources. An inaccurate claim can destroy an advocacy organisation's credibility and give ammunition to opponents, so this must be avoided at all costs (PHAIWA 2013a; Chapman 2007). Advocates should practice using a short list of 'key facts' to support their arguments in different ways for various audiences. Many advocacy organisations gather their own evidence, using polls and surveys about the experiences and opinions of people affected by the issue and/or the proposed policy decision. This is not only a powerful tool for exerting political pressure, but it also ensures that the perspectives of everyday citizens are considered as legitimate evidence used to inform expert decision-making processes (see Chapter 9; also see Freudenberg et al. 2009).

There are multiple opportunities for health practitioners to influence public policy. Within local schools, community organisations and councils, as well as state and national governments, policies are constantly being created and modified in ways that can undermine or enhance health. In fact, health workers, health promotion practitioners and public health researchers have a legitimate and powerful role in ensuring that public policy is developed in ways that enhance health and social equity (Gould et al. 2012). They have a unique position as advocates for public health that combines credibility within communities, access to decision-makers, knowledge of the broad factors influencing health and access to the evidence needed to bring about change. In the following section, we refresh our understanding of policy-making and identify ways to utilise these opportunities for influence.

Healthy public policy: Opportunities for influence

What is healthy public policy?

A policy is a formal statement by an entity which conveys values and a commitment to action. Public policy is made by an appropriate authority to describe important goals, such as national health priorities, 'what' will be done (a statement of intended actions) or 'how' things will be done (a set of rules or codes of conduct). The term 'healthy public policy' refers to public policy in any area or sector which has a positive effect on health and/or social inequity (Baum 2008). Several examples are provided in Table10.2.

Why health is a political issue
Policies are made by governments and organisations and so they imply particular sets of values. Public policies often reflect the values of the decision-makers who develop them – and also those of the interest groups seeking to influence

Table 10.2   Healthy public policy examples

1. Public sector	Health policy: • Universal health care • Pharmaceutical benefits schemes • Public hospitals Social and economic policy: • Social security: economic support and social safety net • Taxation and 'income redistribution' • Workplace: safety regulations, fair payment standards • Education: support schemes for low-income families • Housing: affordable public housing for vulnerable groups • Transport: concessions for public transport • Environment: regulation of harmful industrial practices • Laws and regulations (e.g. traffic safety, tobacco control) • Media and communication: access to community media
2. Private sector	• Workplaces: safe and fair working conditions • Product manufacturers (e.g. food industry labelling of additives, restrictions on trans fats and salt content) • Retailers: marketing and advertising codes of practice (e.g. junk foods to children)
3. Community and volunteers	• Sports clubs: codes of conduct; first-aid training • Community safety committees • School councils: healthy school meals programmes

the policy-making process (Talbot & Verrinder 2014). The strengths and limitations of a particular policy can be viewed differently depending on these values and the broader political ideologies of the government of the day (see Chapter 2).

For example, social justice oriented governments generally pursue policies that aim to create a more equitable distribution of income, wealth and access to secure work, housing and health care. These policies tend to be widely supported by health practitioners and community organisations whose work is underpinned by the principles of primary health care and a social model of health. Conversely, politicians and people who value neoliberal ideology, economic conservatism and individualism have vigorously opposed these policies (Laverack 2013; Baum 2008).

In an example focused on public health nutrition in the United Kingdom and Australia, government policies seeking to regulate television advertising of 'junk' foods to young children have been welcomed by public health professionals. However, they have been vigorously opposed by voters concerned about erosion of civil liberties and by commercial vested interests such as processed food manufacturers and retailers seeking to maximise profit through sales of snack foods (Laverack 2013).

Power and public policy
Public policy is very often about who gets what, when, where and how. Clearly then, policy is also about power. Those with greater access to power, resources and the media have greater capacity to set the agenda and influence public discussion and debate about issues which affect health. In many cases, public policy is actually created to provide checks and balances against the abuse of power – including bullying, coercion, unfair bargaining and manipulative actions (Keleher & MacDougall 2007). To this extent, public policy is profoundly political.

As we noted earlier in this chapter, health professionals and health promotion practitioners have a key role in advocating for healthy public policy. In part, this involves influencing public discussion and shaping debates about the kinds of policies that are likely to make a difference to public health. It is also about becoming actively engaged in the policy-making process in order to influence decision-makers. We will now turn to the policy-making process and the multiple opportunities this creates health practitioners to influence healthy public policy.

The process of policy-making: Opportunities for influence

Policy-making generally follows a cyclic process. This is illustrated in Figure 10.1, along with opportunities for communication to influence in this process. Talbot and Verrinder (2005) have identified five stages in the policy-making cycle: issue identification, policy formation, adoption, implementation and evaluation. Public health advocacy groups, including researchers, practitioners and community members, can influence the process of policy-making at each stage. First, by bringing issues onto the public agenda, including

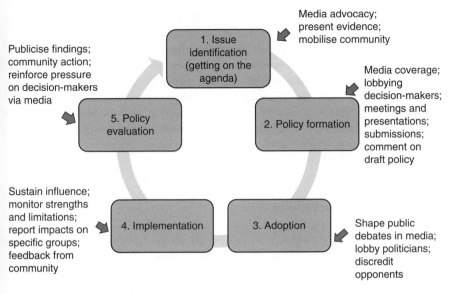

Figure 10.1   Process of policy-making

unrecognised public health issues or those being strategically overlooked by decision-makers. At this stage, advocacy groups must strategically use a diverse mix of media to raise public awareness, present evidence for change and mobilise community support (see also Chapter 9).

During policy formation, advocacy groups make formal, evidence-based submissions to government working parties and they respond to calls for public comment on draft policies. This often involves analysis of existing policies and presenting the case for what change is needed. They may also lobby politicians directly, seeking personal meetings and giving presentations at formal hearings. Community forums are often conducted to draw various stakeholders together and ensure that the views of community members affected by the issue are represented. This stage provides valuable opportunities to secure media coverage to increase pressure on decision-makers (Ricketts 2012).

The next stage, 'adoption', is critical because this is involves pushing the policy forward and deciding whether or not it should be adopted. This stage usually involves decision-makers weighing up the arguments from supporters and opponents. Public health advocacy coalitions and alliances have a pivotal role here, in shaping public debates through the media and directly lobbying politicians and government. This is a critical stage because it aims to secure wider political support from a broader range of relevant decision-makers. This involves convincing decision-makers in other departments and sectors of government, including those who control finances and budgets, to support the adoption of a healthy public policy (Laverack 2013).

During the implementation phase, advocacy groups undertake research (or synthesise research by others) to monitor the strengths and limitations of the policy and particularly its impacts on specific communities or population groups. Community groups themselves are an important source of evidence, gathering their own data through surveys within their communities and presenting personal stories (Brown et al. 2004a). The media provides an important conduit for engaging communities in this process, publicising community activism and ensuring the politicians respond to community calls for action (see Chapter 9). At the review stage, public health advocates commonly pressure decision-makers by using the media to draw attention to these findings and present formal evidence to argue why the policy should be maintained and/or amended (Ricketts 2012).

How advocacy works in practice

In practice, advocacy works at a number of levels. In addition to their role as direct participants in the policy-making process, health practitioners also engage in advocacy to influence the people whom Ricketts (2012) refers to as 'power-holders'. These are the people with decision-making power and also the people who have a wider influence on their decisions.

Targets audiences for advocacy

Public health advocacy uses a variety of media and communication strategies to target those individuals and organisations with the power to influence policies, practices or living and/or working conditions. Primary target audiences are those with decision-making power. Secondary audiences are those with the power to influence decision-makers. Importantly, as we discussed in Chapter 2 (see the Cultural Model of media and communication), these 'audiences' are also actively engaged as 'producers' of media content with the potential to have a considerable influence on decision-makers. As we illustrate in chapters 6, 7 and 9, this has a pivotal role to play in effective advocacy.

Primary target audiences

The primary target audiences most commonly involve the 'public sector'. These are the decision-makers responsible for changing or maintaining laws, regulations and public policies that have implications for almost every aspect of society. Public sector policy-makers include members of government (local, state, provincial or national) and public service administrators (including various funding agencies, programme managers, regulatory bodies, boards of appeal, tribunals and courts).

These are important audiences for advocacy because they can, for example:

- change or propose new laws or regulations (such as regulations on advertising junk food during children's peak TV viewing times);
- take action to ensure laws and industry regulations are better enforced (such as legal action against a corporation using deceptive marketing);

- change policy about procedures, safeguards, guidelines and practice (such as food labelling, removing confectionery food from supermarket checkouts, standards for provision of healthy foods in childcare and education settings);
- withdraw programme funding and reallocate it to more effective public health initiatives (such as health-promoting school canteens, community gardens, facilities for active play, cycle trails and public transport);
- support public health research programmes (to build the evidence-base on the effectiveness of public health interventions); and
- use this evidence to convince other decision-makers (to allocate a greater share of 'health' funding to public health and prevention initiatives).

Secondary target audiences

Secondary target audiences are those with the power to *influence* decision-makers. These are the groups, leaders and community members who see themselves as stakeholders in the issue. It is essential to reach these audiences as they have an important role as potential advocates and change agents (Green & Tones 2010). Some examples of audiences are provided in Table 10.3

The private sector. The private sector has had a substantial influence on government policy-making over recent decades as corporations have grown larger, more economically powerful and therefore increasingly able to exert influence on government policy decisions and political processes (Laverack 2013). Reciprocally, many of the government policy changes sought by public health advocacy aim to influence corporate practices, as we saw in both earlier case studies.

While private sector opposition to public health initiatives is a legitimate cause for concern amongst many advocacy groups (see Chapter 9), it should

Table 10.3   Target audiences for advocacy

Public sector	Social and community services, health practitioners and researchers
	Opposition politicians who are not members of government and therefore capable of exercising considerable critical pressure on the govenment of the day
Private sector	Private providers of health and other support services in the community
	Employers (and employees) in privately controlled, profit-making businesses
	Executives in large corporations and their shareholders
	Influential business leaders and industry bodies
Civil society	Community groups and opinion leaders, such as those in:

- patient support and consumer advocacy groups
- parents groups, school councils and other educational institutions
- religious and cultural organisations
- political parties, unions and worker's organisations
- charities and not-for-profit organisations

also be remembered that the private sector can also provide valuable allies. Small, locally based private enterprise can often be strong supporters of action to create more health promoting social and physical environments in local communities. After all, healthy, vibrant and cohesive communities with low levels of crime and violence, good public transport and employment opportunities are in their best interests. To this extent, they can be an important positive influence on political decision-makers and are therefore a key secondary audience for public health advocacy campaigns (Ricketts 2012).

Civil society groups. Civil society interest groups concerned about inequalities, social justice and environmental issues tend to share common goals with those of public health. These are often the people who are most easily mobilised to apply political pressure for policy changes to address the underlying causes of ill-health (Laverack 2013). Importantly, many of these groups have a philanthropic dimension to their activities. They can be a great source of funding and in-kind support, such as access to office space, equipment, media relations experience, volunteers and even some level of funding to support the advocacy campaign until change is achieved.

Securing the political support of civil society groups relies on the communication skills of advocates in presenting their case in a compelling way that ties into the values and mission of the organisation. It also helps to provide opportunities for people's participation in the advocacy process.

Ambassadors and champions. Many civil society groups have some association with high-profile individuals, such as important cultural leaders, celebrities and former politicians, who can *leverage* greater political influence through their existing networks, media contacts and/or public notoriety. Individuals with highly regarded professional expertise or powerful connections can also gain political leverage. They may be interested in *championing the cause* for an advocacy campaign. Community groups can help advocates to access people affected by the issue (and their families or carers) become *ambassadors*. These are people willing to speak publicly about their own experiences and perspectives on the problem in ways that support the proposed policy solution (see Summer Foundation 2012).

Strategies for advocacy

Public health advocacy achieves its goals through a combination of communication strategies designed to gain political commitment for change. According to Chapman (2007), the three most important advocacy strategies are political lobbying, media advocacy and building coalitions for community action.

- **Political lobbying** uses direct communication with decision-makers to present the case for change and influence the policy process.
- **Coalitions and alliances** involving community groups, professional and other key stakeholders committed to organising community action and maintaining public pressure on decision-makers.

- **Media advocacy** works with the media to set the agenda, shape public debates, discredit the opposition and advance policy development.

In the next sections, we will discuss each of these strategies separately, along with important considerations for communication and utilising various forms of media.

Political lobbying: Working with decision-makers

Political lobbying is a strategy for working with governments and politicians to influence policy-making. Lobbying refers to the direct communication between advocates and a government decision-maker. In most democratic systems, lobbying is an everyday part of the political process. According to Laverack (2013: 120),

> lobbyists commonly describe themselves as forming a bridge between government and the governed, across which information can flow in order to ensure that policy decisions are better informed and that people can interact with policymakers more frequently. Policymakers also find it useful to be provided with information by lobbyists about the possible impact of a policy decision.

How to identify the decision-makers

Lobbying is most effective when it targets the right decision-makers. That is, the people with power to make decisions about the issue and/or particular solution that the lobbyists are proposing. The following four questions are a helpful guide to identifying the right targets for lobbying.

1. What is the policy decision being sought?
2. Which level of government (local, state or national) holds responsibility for the issue and proposed solution?
3. At this level, which departments or portfolio areas are stakeholders? Most public health issues involve several portfolio areas. For example, a proposal for safer cycling lanes could involve portfolios of health, transport, education, housing, policing and security.
4. What opportunities exist for working with all sides of government, including opposition politicians and minor political parties? (PHAIWA 2013a).

Public health advocates commonly lobby decision-makers who already have an existing interest in the issue and/or who are already sympathetic to their position. This is far more likely to achieve change than trying to convince someone who holds strong opposing views. Politicians and government representatives in marginal electorates are also good targets, particularly if they believe that supporting your position could win them important votes or a seat in government (Ricketts 2012). Opposition politicians are often willing to support innovative public health policy initiatives. Although they do not necessarily have responsibility for their implementation, they are capable of exercising considerable critical pressure on the government of the day (Ricketts 2012). The powerful importance of lobbying opponents is illustrated in the following example.

Lobbying potential opponents: Every Australian counts
In Australia, when a groundbreaking, comprehensive national disability insurance scheme, *Disability Care*, was being considered by parliament in 2012, the Every Australian Counts advocacy campaign made sure they targeted both the government and leader of the opposition, Tony Abbott. With a federal election looming, and recognising the potential electoral advantage, the usually conservative Abbott claimed he would implement the innovative scheme if elected. This helped to ensure the bill was passed in parliament with strong support from all parties. Soon afterwards, the incumbent Labour government lost the election. Abbott was elected as the Prime Minister and his new government had little choice but to follow through with their electoral promise to fund the rollout of the scheme (Every Australian Counts 2013).

Building relationships: Working with government and politicians

Gaining political commitment for change involves advocacy groups building relationships with the decision-makers they are seeking to influence. Advocates can develop opportunities to work closely with decision-makers by maintaining good communication, building mutual respect and trust and being a source of reliable evidence-based information (Reber & Kim 2006; also see Chapter 9, Health Activism).

Advocates can help decision-makers to do their job by keeping them informed and by providing compelling arguments for change that are consistent with the existing priorities and policy decisions of their department or agency. Getting to know their political interests and personal views is particularly important (Parvanta et al. 2011). These relationships can help public health advocates to negotiate a win-win outcome with decision-makers without the issue 'going public'. Many decision-makers prefer this approach because it enables them to maintain a sense of controlling the agenda rather than responding to community complaints, protest or potentially damaging public controversy.

Lobbying tools
Advocates use a range of tools for lobbying government and politicians. These include activities are categorised by Ontario HP Resource System (Johnson 2009) as follows. *Low-profile activities*: quiet negotiation, meetings with public service bureaucrats, providing research evidence and other key information, development of an in-house briefing paper. *Medium-profile activities*: public briefing papers, negotiation via participation on committees and working parties, writing letters to politicians, meeting with elected officials, forming strategic alliances with other groups, writing letters to newspapers, media

advocacy. *High profile*: presenting to formal commissions and inquiries, organ-ising professional conferences and public forums to which politicians are invited, news and current affairs interviews, advertising campaigns.

Working at a local level: Advocacy in local communities

Evidence from around the world indicates that local advocacy campaigns on local issues driven by local communities are more effective in changing govern-ments and corporate practices than those attempting change at a national or global scale (Freudenberg et al. 2009). According to Ricketts (2012) most gov-ernment policy change occurs through a series of small wins, beginning with change at the local government level and gathering momentum and public support for more widespread policy change. Local governments rely on grass-roots support and their representatives are easier to access. They are often closely engaged with a range of community groups and local businesses and therefore in a good position to raise awareness of the issue and generate public support for the proposed solution, including promoting ways for people to get involved.

Practical tips for local lobbying
Common tools for lobbying decision-makers include letter writing, personal meetings with politicians and making formal presentations. Each of these communication strategies relies upon advocates' capacity to develop their arguments into a compelling and persuasive case for change that will appeal to local decision-makers. It is important to present wider public health issues in terms of their prevalence, causes and small-scale solutions at a local level. Provide statistics for the issue gathered locally. Outline how the issue affects local community members. Involve a local spokesperson (PHAIWA 2013a).

Ranking and score cards.   Report cards are a highly effective way to present data about how their locality measures up in comparison with others. The powerful importance of this approach is illustrated in the following example from Colombia. An advocacy campaign seeking support for universal immu-nisation sent each local government candidate a report card specific to their electorate with statistics about current vaccination rates and the local incidence of illnesses that it could prevent. Graphics were used to show how the perfor-mance of their electorate was ranked in comparison to the others. The package was accompanied by a personal letter from a child, telling the candidate about the problem and asking, 'Mayoral candidate, what can you do for me? Will you help me?' Posters of the child and her key message were posted throughout the community to ensure the issue remained in the public eye – and on political agenda. The campaign was specifically tailored for each local government area, engaging communities in the process of lobbying local decision-makers. It was spectacularly successful in increasing immunisation rates across the country (Singhal 2011).

More generally, arguments for policy change should also identify under-lying causes of the issue that are relevant to the specific community. Use a

combination of quantitative and qualitative evidence. Quantitative population data provides decision-makers with useful empirical facts. Qualitative
research is useful for presenting the personal experiences and perspectives
of local people on this issue and what they think about the proposed
initiative.

Propose initial solutions that are small, low-cost and easy to implement
so that local decision-makers can demonstrate progress to the community.
Demonstrate how small achievements can win public support and build
momentum for wider change. Use evidence about success stories in other
localities. If evidence isn't yet available, perhaps another local government is
trialling the same intervention? Friendly competition between local government areas is not uncommon and can also be a good motivator for bureaucrats
and practitioners to adopt new initiatives (Singhal 2011).

Examples and further practical tips for effectively presenting these arguments through letter writing, presentations and meetings with government
departments and politicians, can be found in the *Advocacy in Action
Toolkit* (PHAIWA 2013a) and in practical handbooks by Ricketts (2012) and
Shaw (2013).

Coalitions and alliances: Building momentum for change

As we noted in Chapter 9, most social change has been brought about
through organised groups of people working collectively. One of the most
effective ways to build capacity for political influence is by forming larger
coalitions and alliances that can create a sustained political presence. Most
public health advocacy coalitions involve community groups, health professionals, experts and other stakeholder groups who are committed to maintaining public pressure on decision-makers in government and corporations
(Laverack 2013).

National coalition for gun control

The National Coalition for Gun Control, for example, is a coalition of associations and individuals committed to tightening the regulation of guns in order to
reduce gun-related community violence in Australia. Over 300 organisations
have supported NCGC from the fields of public health, medicine, law, domestic violence advocacy, women's, religious, ethnic and community groups. The
coalition was instrumental in achieving the landmark 1996 gun control laws
and continues to maintain pressure on governments to counteract the influence
of the powerful gun lobby, to ensure stringent gun laws are not undermined
and to further advance gun control policy (Chapman 2013).

Advocacy coalitions often work in partnership with existing community
activist organisations and their networks of pressure groups, drawing on
their capacity to mobilise large numbers of people and organise widespread
community action in support of a cause (see Chapter 9).

The Parents Jury

The Parents Jury is an online network of parents, grandparents and guardians, who are interested in improving the food and physical activity environments of children in Australia. The Parents Jury was formed in 2004 with the goal of maintaining a strong and sustained political presence on a range of issues affecting children – and to provide a political voice for concerned community members.

Thousands of members are regularly mobilised through online surveys, opinion polls, petitions, email letter campaigns and events. The Parent Jury has forcefully advocated to governments to influence their election priorities, and it has campaigned for changes to food labelling, unhealthy promotions and sports sponsorship and healthy school canteens. The network is supported by peak national organisations focused on the prevention of cancer, diabetes and obesity (Parents Jury 2013). For more information, go to www.parentsjury. org.au.

Most healthy public policies involve a range of sectors other than health. By forging strategic connections with other sectors with overlapping interests, advocacy coalitions are able to strengthen their legitimacy and achieve greater success. As the case studies in this chapter have illustrated, working on shared agendas provides opportunities to mobilise a larger base of supporters, share knowledge and resources and build on the past success of other advocacy organisations (Freudenberg et al. 2009). Furthermore, coalitions can help to secure media coverage of the advocacy campaign and key issues. Journalists seek reliable sources of expert opinion and convincing and reliable evidence, as well as access to respected spokespersons and community members. Well-established coalitions place advocates in a better position to support the needs of journalists and build positive, ongoing relationships with media professionals (Reber & Kim 2006).

Action on Smoking and Health

Action on Smoking and Health (ASH) is an international alliance of interest groups working in over 100 countries to advance tobacco control policies at local and global levels. ASH aims to build alliances and coalitions with capacity to influence governments, politicians and corporate practices. These coalitions involve public health, legal and medical experts in partnership with other sectors including child protection, human rights, environment and workers organisations.

ASH coalitions have been highly effective in using media advocacy to educate the public and decision-makers in government and the private sector. They have successfully campaigned for policy initiatives in many countries. In the United States, ASH provides legal assistance to assist coalition members exert legal pressure for change (ASH 2013). In partnership with the World Health Organisation, ASH monitors the strategies used by the tobacco industry to systematically undermine strong tobacco control policies and make this evidence publicly available (WHO 2012). In the United Kingdom, ASH Scotland coordinates a host of publications, research documents, evidence-based briefings and advocacy resources for tobacco control that are used by advocates around the world (ASH Scotland 2013).

Changing health-damaging corporate practices

Each of the above case studies illustrates the power of coalitions to influence government policy and, ultimately, corporate practices that damage health. Freudenberg et al. (2009) have analysed case studies of advocacy to change corporate practices in the alcohol, automobile, food and beverage, firearms, pharmaceutical and tobacco industries. The most effective campaigns included a mix of formal advocacy (to influence public policy) and community activism (to mobilise community action from consumers and shareholders). Other success factors included

- involving diverse constituencies;
- framing the campaign in terms of fairness and social justice;
- starting at a local level to influence one company; and
- linking many small campaigns that, together, have a cumulative effect on the practices of health-damaging industries.

These features are demonstrated in the highly successful international alliance, *Corporate Accountability International*, involving tens of thousands of members around the world working on bold campaigns to protect human rights, public health and the environment from corporate greed and abuse. Readers interested in their strategies and tactics will find a wealth of inspiring examples and success stories at http://www.stopcorporateabuse.org/.

Media advocacy: Making news

Media advocacy primarily involves interventions in news reporting and 'aims to shift the ways in which communities and issues are reported, framed and defined' (Dreher 2010). It is defined by Chapman (2004: 361) as the 'strategic use of news media to advance a policy initiative, often in the face of highly organised opposition'. More specifically, it involves working with the media to set the agenda, shape public debates, discredit the opposition and influence policy decisions (The Health Communication Unit (THCU) 2000).

Politicians and the wider public routinely identify news and current affairs as their key source of information about health issues (Chapman et al. 2009). News media have a powerful role in setting the public and policy agenda. They are also instrumental to the process of defining public health 'problems' and framing proposed solutions. News stories provide unrivalled opportunities for framing health issues in ways that build support for healthy public policy. Public health advocacy organisations use media advocacy to 'make full use of news channels by reacting to news and creating it. They present themselves as partners in the news-making and gathering processes' (Green & Tones 2010: 391).

Framing public health issues

Framing refers to the way an issue is presented. It is a process whereby some aspects of a perceived reality are made salient in a way which promotes a particular problem definition, causal interpretation, moral evaluation, and/or recommendation for action (Chapman 2007). Framing is important because it has a significant impact on what policy solutions are considered feasible and who should be involved in creating those solutions.

Reframing and how it works

As we noted in Chapter 4, news media tend to frame health issues in terms of individual responsibility and behavioural and/or medical solutions. Media advocacy seeks to 'reframe' a particular health issue to emphasise the need for social accountability, shifting the focus from individual responsibility to the social and environmental causes, and presenting a clear policy solution.

Reframing is also used discredit the arguments of those opposing a policy initiative. This often involves shifting a 'negative' frame to a more 'positive' one. For example, the tobacco industry and tobacco control advocates frame the same issue in very different ways in order to shape public opinion and influence decision-makers. The tobacco industry frames 'tobacco control' in terms of censorship, discrimination against smokers, removing people's right to choose, restrictions on fair trading and undermining a legitimate agricultural industry. Tobacco control advocates, on the other hand, frame the issue in terms of child protection; civil liberties and the right to breathe uncontaminated air; and freedom from pervasive marketing of an addictive drug. Tobacco is reframed as a lethal product and the tobacco industry is portrayed as irresponsible, deceptive, manipulative and unethical (THCU 2000).

This process of reframing clearly identifies the 'problem' as the tobacco industry and the 'solution' becomes stronger regulation and policies to protect consumers. The 'target for change' shifts from individual smokers to decision-makers in government and powerful multinational tobacco corporations.

Evidence, emotions and values

Successful media advocacy presents compelling data and evidence-based arguments. However, evidence alone is not enough to change the minds of intransigent decision-makers (Chapman 2007). Advocates need to engage the emotions of audiences through creative rhetorical strategies that involve framing problems and their policy solutions in ways that appeal to commonly held public interest values. These might include fairness, freedom, democracy, security, financial responsibility, social justice and/or environmental sustainability. Advocates often draw upon widely held ethical concerns, such as vulnerability, protection of children, human rights, abuses of power and deceitful or dishonest behaviour (THCU 2000).

Framing the main message involves four key steps outline by Johnson (2009):

1. emphasising the social dimensions of the problem;
2. shifting primary responsibility away from the affected individuals to those whose decisions affect these conditions;
3. presenting policy alternatives as solutions; and
4. ensuring that policy options have practical appeal.

Making the news: Understanding the news-making process

News, current affairs and feature stories in print, radio, television and online media provide many opportunities for advocacy groups to influence public discussion and political debate. Advocacy organisations can work with the media proactively or in a responsive manner. *Working proactively* involves developing rapport with media professionals and approaching the media for coverage. *Working responsively* involves responding to media requests (for expert information or comment about an issue) or by responding to news media stories (about issues relevant to the advocacy organisation) (Mindframe Media 2011).

In order to attract the interest of news media journalists, it is essential to understand a little about the news-making process and the constraints that journalists face as part of everyday news-making routines and timeframes. The contemporary 'news cycle' involves the media reporting on a story, followed by further media reporting on public and other reactions to earlier reports. Online and cable news have quickened the pace of this process, creating increasing demand for stories that can be followed and continually updated.

Within this increasingly competitive news media environment (see Chapter 4), journalists are constrained by substantial time pressure to produce more stories in limited space – either lines of text or time on air. The drive to produce 'more with less' has meant that news is rarely 'gathered'. In fact, the vast majority of news stories are sourced directly from media releases and other public relations materials provided by influential organisations, government bodies and corporate interests (Waldman 2011).

Only a small proportion of this material is selected and used as the basis for stories. Public health advocates must therefore be extremely strategic if they are to compete for coverage. The first step involves seeding a story in the media and ensuring that it gets picked up. Once a news story is covered, different media outlets then feed off each other, competing to provide various 'new' angles on the story, more in-depth analysis and critique. Blogs, wikis and other social media provide valuable opportunities for initiating stories that are then picked up by mainstream media. They are also highly effective for circulating and sharing related stories, generating wider public comment and feeding into community and political debates in mainstream media (see Chapter 9).

News triggers and ongoing themes
According to research by Chapman and colleagues (2009), The most common 'triggers' for health-related news stories to be incident-based 'hard' news

(42%), research (11%), celebrity illness (10%) and new treatments and trials (10%). Health news stories last a median duration of 97 seconds and feature only two news 'actors' (spokespeople), with up to four actors in current affairs stories. Sound bite duration was between seven and nine seconds respectively.

This 'episodic' reporting affords journalists little opportunity for reconstructing complex public health issues as accessible stories for general audiences. On the other hand, journalists also develop 'thematic' stories that place the issue within its larger social and political context and create the potential for ongoing coverage and related, incident-based stories. For this to be possible within contemporary news-making, journalists need to rely on established sources: reliable contacts who can provide 'jargon-free' technical information, credible experts and access to interest groups willing to be interview participants (Reber & Kim 2006).

Approaching the media: Developing media relations

Good relationships with news journalists are therefore essential for public health advocacy. Before approaching the media for coverage, it is important to be well prepared. Several excellent practical guides for developing good media relations include Mindframe Media (2011), PHAIWA (2013a) and Ricketts (2012). Below, we provide a selection of practical tips for developing good media relations.

Plan ahead
Before you approach the media, be very clear about the following:

- WHAT you want to say (what messages do you want to communicate?)
- WHO you are saying it to (what audience/s do you want to reach?)
- WHERE AND WHEN you want to say it (how will you access each audience?)
- WHY you want to say it (what outcomes are you seeking?)

Build relationships
Find out about the media organisation: editors, relevant journalists, schedules. Make personal contact, introduce yourself and establish your credibility. Provide information about your organisation: mission statement, who is involved, goals and objectives, how you aim to achieve these. Get to know relevant production schedules, deadlines, bad days or times. Respect the expertise of the journalist and always express appreciation.

Be a reliable source
Establish your organisation's capacity to be a source of expert opinion, accurate current evidence, respected spokespersons and relevant community members. Be available: always respond to journalists' enquiries.

Develop and maintain a website
A website is instrumental for cultivating mutually beneficial media relationships between advocacy organisations and media professionals (Reber & Kim 2006). The website should meet the needs of busy journalists, making it easier for them to cover issues of interest to the advocacy organisation. In Chapter 9, we describe the essential features of these websites from the perspective of journalists and public relations experts.

Getting news stories selected

News values
Stories are selected according to their 'newsworthy' qualities so advocates need to consider the news angle they will adopt and how to 'pitch' the story in a newsworthy way. While an 'issue' may be important, this is not enough to ensure it gets coverage. For example, the issue of excessive drinking is not itself newsworthy, but when a football star is unconscious in hospital after trying to break up a drunken pub brawl, that's a story likely to make the news. It also provides the springboard for advocates to present the case for public health approaches to the problem.

Criteria for newsworthiness are often referred to as 'news values'. They include:

- CURRENCY: link the story to recent news or events; highlight new information about an existing issue; introduce important, different voices to debates; introduce compelling facts and new perspectives to change focus of debate;
- CONSEQUENCE: show how the issue affects many people, or few people but with dramatic effects;
- CLOSENESS: highlight aspects of the issue occurring in local area or involving a local person;
- NOVELTY: draw attention to a bizarre, unexpected or extraordinary person or event;
- PROMINENCE: create links with a high profile organisation, person, or celebrity; use 'piggybacking' to build on an issue or government policy currently prominent in the news;
- HUMAN INTEREST: convey a personal story; someone affected by this issue;
- CONFLICT: highlight controversy, such as competing views about the 'problem' and/or what solution is best; expose unexpected tensions and disagreements; draw attention to protests and other forms of opposition (Chapman 2007; Chapman & Lupton 1994).

The news angle
News values help to draw out what is currently newsworthy about the issue. The most salient of these is then selected and developed to create the news 'angle'. This is used to attract the attention of journalists via a strategically targeted media release (see later). Advocacy groups often develop several different

angles, with a corresponding media release, so the same issue/story can be pitched in an appropriate way for each media outlet and the audience they are trying to reach (Mindframe Media 2011).

As we noted earlier in this chapter, advocates may take either a proactive approach (pitching a potential story to the media) or a reactive approach (responding to an existing media story, event or issue). A common strategy involves advocacy groups generating their 'own' newsworthy activities such as releasing a report, or launching a public forum, new campaign or community event. The newsworthiness of these events can be considerably heightened by taking 'news values' into account in the planning stages, for example, by involving a politician, celebrity or important cultural figure in a key role.

Opportunities for newsworthy stories can also be created by community action and activism groups through public rallies, protests, publicity stunts and various forms of online grass-roots action. As we noted in Chapter 9, it is common practice for community action groups to develop an online presence, strategically creating campaign websites and utilizing e-petitions, YouTube, blogs and a range of social media. Not only are these media highly effective for organizing targeted action by large numbers of people, they also provide a rich source of material for journalist's stories. Strategies for working with community action groups and more health activists to generate media coverage are covered extensively in Chapter 9.

In summary, media advocacy involves public health advocates engaging with and creating news stories. Advocates can become more effective agents of change by shifting their focus from simply talking about the social, economic, political causes of health problems towards a more strategic approach incorporating news values, framing, proactive and reactive approaches and partnerships with media professionals.

How to plan an advocacy campaign

In this final section of the chapter, we focus on the practical steps involved in planning an advocacy campaign. We illustrate this with a recent case study that tells the story of a passionately committed group of people involved in an ongoing advocacy campaign to get young people out of nursing homes.

Summer Foundation: Building better lives for young people in nursing homes

When Ben Thompson was 22 years old, he acquired a brain injury as a result of an unprovoked attack. After surgery and an initial stay in hospital, Ben spent more than three years living in a nursing home. He had very few visits from friends and spent most of his time in a small room. He didn't talk, could only communicate through an electronic device and was fed through a tube. It was only when Ben moved out of the nursing home that he started talking, eating and gradually restoring his quality of life. Getting young people out of nursing homes is essential in helping them recover and reach their potential. Michelle Newland acquired a brain injury after a near-fatal asthma attack just after she finished high school. She lived in a nursing home for 18 months but now, after many years of rehabilitation, she has the support she needs to live in the community, and she works as a public speaker and assistant in a primary school. For Sarah Ryan, a debilitating stroke caused her brain injury when her baby was three months old. Without other options for her care, she lived in a nursing home for six months. Several years later, she was able to walk a 5-kilometre fund-raising run with 60 others wearing T-shirts with the slogan 'I'm taking steps to get young people out of nursing homes!'

Summer Foundation is a non-profit organisation focused on building better lives for young people in nursing homes. In Australia in 2012, there were more than 600 young people with complex care needs living in nursing homes where the average age is 84 years. The goal of Summer Foundation is to stop young people being forced into nursing homes simply because there is nowhere else for them to go. Since 2006, Summer Foundation has been passionately committed to this issue, led by occupational therapist, Di Winkler, and a growing team of health practitioners, other professionals and volunteers. The mission of the Summer Foundation is to develop an integrated housing model for young people with disability and persuade decision-makers of its potential to resolve the issue of young people living in nursing homes in Australia. They use a three-way advocacy approach shown in Figure 10.2. This involves research, creating a movement and demonstrating evidence for alternative housing options.

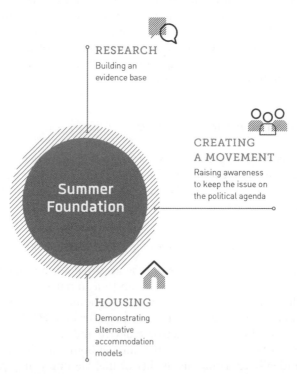

Figure 10.2   Summer Foundation: Three-way advocacy approach

Source: Summer Foundation (2013)

1. *Research*

Summer Foundation conduct and foster research to provide the evidence base for policy change. The research demonstrates the impact of inappropriate living environments on young people, identifies interventions to improve their lives, documents the outcomes of providing supported housing options and establishes the economic benefits of alternatives to nursing home care. By publicising research and stories about the changed lives of young people who have moved out of nursing homes, they demonstrate the potential for improving quality of life for young people and their families – and the critical importance of creating pathways back into community living.

In order to influence policy, Summer Foundation presents this research in accessible ways through direct meetings with key government representatives and submissions to policy-makers and funders, conference presentations, formal reports and print, and radio and television media outlets.

2. *Creating a movement*

Summer Foundation clearly identifies the issue of concern: young people should not be forced to live in nursing homes because there is nowhere else for them. The solutions they propose include (i) more accessible and affordable housing and (ii) support services to prevent new admissions by helping young people demonstrate their potential for independent living.

Using the advocacy slogan, 'Building better lives for young people in nursing homes', Summer Foundation aims to raise awareness, generate public support and keep the issue on the political agenda. In particular, they provide support for young people with a disability to tell their personal stories about living in a nursing home and/or returning to supported living in the community. Their 'ambassador' programme provides these young people with training and support to create their own digital stories and share them through print media, radio and television, social media and speaking engagements with community and corporate audiences. These are available on the Summer Foundation YouTube channel.

'Tell Your Story' workshops conducted around the country create opportunities for more young people to capture, document and record their experiences of living in a nursing home, finding alternatives and returning to community life. Their public exhibitions, Home to Home, present short films, written stories and photos to invite politicians, media and a wide public audience.

Summer Foundation ambassadors are inspirational young people who are making a significant contribution to systemic advocacy by telling and retelling their often heart-breaking stories. When an ambassador shares his or her story, the dire situation of young people in nursing homes is powerfully communicated.

For Summer Foundation, social media continue to be central to the process of enhancing linkages between people and communities with an interest in this issue. By providing online spaces for sharing stories, knowledge and resources, new opportunities are being created for bringing people together and mobilising community action. The social media links on the organisation's home page (www.summerfoundation.org) help to facilitate support between people and organisations trying to generate social and political change (Plate 10.1).

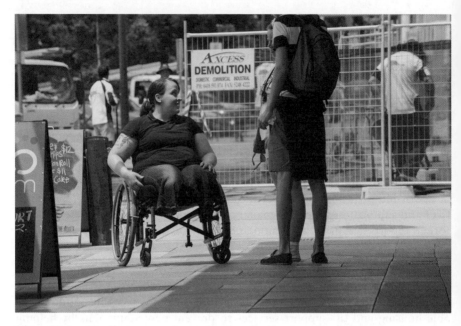

Plate 10.1   Kirrily is an ambassador for the Summer Foundation, raising community awareness about getting young people out of nursing homes

Source: Summer Foundation

3. *Demonstrating alternative housing options*

The advocacy work of Summer Foundation has been pivotal in securing funding to develop, trial and evaluate several innovative models of housing so that more young people with disability can be moved out of nursing homes.

Summer Foundation aims to demonstrate that by providing good-quality housing for young people with disability, this will increase their independence, decrease reliance on paid supports and decrease life-time care costs. Their research is building the evidence base about the benefits of housing that is not segregated, but, instead, is integrated with larger mixed private and social housing developments and has 24-hour on-call support; is centrally located close to public transport and accessible shops in order to reduce transport costs; and is designed to include smart home technology that enables residents to use their iPad or smartphone to control lighting, blinds, cooling and heating, external doors and doorbell functions, as well as contacting support staff when needed.

In 2013, the Australian government and several private organisations committed funding to help establish the first of these demonstration housing projects, with the intention that young people would move in shortly after their completion.

In summary, Summer Foundation utilises each of the three key advocacy strategies outlined earlier in this chapter: political lobbying, media advocacy and alliances with a range of non-profit and private sector organisations. They collaborate with researchers, people with disabilities and their families to influence health, housing and disability services policy and practices. Together, they are changing the lives of young people in nursing homes (Summer Foundation 2013, 2012). Further details of Summer Foundation's advocacy materials, such as submission to government, reports, short films and personal stories and media advocacy materials, can be found at https://www.summerfoundation.org.au/ (Figure 10.3)

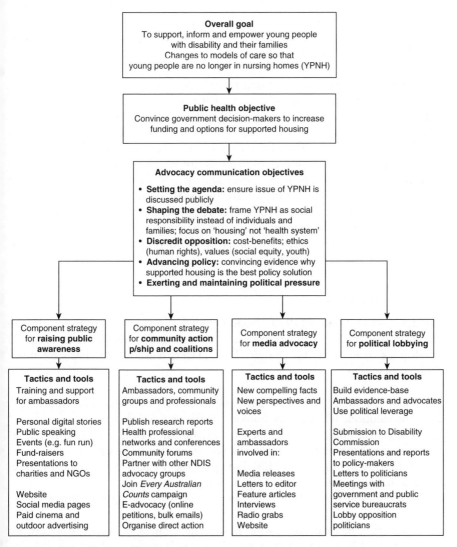

Figure 10.3 Advocacy strategy overview: Building better lives for young people nursing homes (YPNH)

Source: Adapted from Ricketts (2012: 52)

An overview of the advocacy strategies utilised by Summer Foundation is provided in Figure 10.3. This diagram illustrates the relationship between the organisation's goals and objectives, and the strategies, tactics and tools used to achieve these objectives. In the next section, we will take a more detailed look at the process of planning an advocacy strategy.

Strategy planning: The key to effective advocacy

Strategy is the key to effective advocacy because it helps to provide a pathway for the overall campaign. While there are many different approaches to advocacy planning (see PHAIWA 2013a; Chapman 2007; THCU 2000; Wallack et al. 1999), Figure 10.3 provides an example of one simple framework for an integrated strategy plan (Ricketts 2012).

Public health advocacy planning models generally have several key stages in common. The aim of the advocacy plan is to ensure that there is a logical link between the health issue or problem; the causes of the problem; and the goals, objectives and strategies for achieving the policy changes that will help to address them. *Goals* are statements about the long-term benefits or changes the campaign seeks to achieve. *Objectives* are statements of change designed to achieve the goals. They more direct and specific than goals and are linked to immediate outcomes. *Strategies* are the methods that are used or actions that will be taken to achieve these objectives (Keleher 2007). Below, we briefly discuss the following key stages: creating a shared vision, developing the objectives, building evidence-based arguments, identifying the campaign message and designing the media strategy.

Creating a shared vision

Wallack and colleagues (1999) recommend that advocacy groups begin the planning process by brainstorming the following five questions in order to develop a shared vision for change. The answers will form the basis for more detailed planning.

1. The issue: What is the problem (and its causes) and why is it important?
2. The solution: What policy outcome is the group seeking?
3. The power-holders: Which person, organisation or government decision-maker has the power to make the necessary change possible?
4. Action: Who must be mobilised to apply the pressure for change, and how can people get involved or take action?
5. What message would convince those with power to act for change?

It is essential to be clear about what policy change is to be proposed. Decision-making should be informed by available research evidence about what policy approaches have been trialled and evaluated; what factors increase the likelihood of success; and what lesson have been learned that could be applied in this particular context (Ricketts 2012).

From here, the next step is to refine the plan by developing more specific *objectives* and decide on the component *strategies* that will enable the group to achieve these objectives.

Developing objectives

According to Chapman (2007) and Wallack et al. (1999), the advocacy plan requires two distinct sets of objectives: public health objectives and communication objectives.

Public health objectives

It is important to be clear about the specific public health objective (policy change) that will help to achieve the long-term goal of the advocacy campaign. These objectives may include:

* new laws and regulations, or changes to those currently in place;
* enforcement of existing laws and regulations, including stronger penalties;
* more funding for a programme or service;
* tax rises or reductions on products to depress or increase demand;
* changing clinical or institutional practices; or
* having other sectors direct energy at health issues (Chapman 2007).

Consistent with all health promotion planning models, the public health objective(s) should be SMART: Specific, Measurable, Achievable, Realistic and Time-limited. It is important to clearly document the specific change the campaign is seeking. Decide how progress towards the objectives can be measured. Is the objective achievable and realistic, given the timeframes and resources you have available? Advocates should be mindful that small wins can be very valuable so, even if the campaign falls short of achieving the final public health goal, progress towards these objectives is still a significant step forward (PHAIWA 2013a).

Advocacy objectives

Specific objectives should also be set for the advocacy process itself. Also referred to as 'communication objectives', these can be organised as being immediate, short term, intermediate and long term. Examples drawn from THCU (2000) and Chapman (2007) are provided in Table 10.4 along with component strategies to help achieve these objectives.

Building evidence-based arguments

The five planning questions used to develop a shared vision can now be used to help the advocacy group to gather the necessary information to develop the arguments will that underpin the advocacy strategies. The arguments should be well researched, underpinned by accurate and reliable evidence and supported with brief but compelling facts.

Table 10.4 Advocacy communication objectives

Communication objective	Strategies to achieve the objective
Immediate	
Increase media coverage	
Short term	
Setting the agenda	Ensure the issue is publicly discussed
Shaping the debate	Ensure the issue is discussed differently
	Reframe the problem. Outline the policy solution
	Identify the organisation, government department, or individual responsible for making decisions
	Change the focus of a debate by introducing new perspectives and compelling facts
	Introduce important, different voices to debates
Discredit the opposition	Identify and discredit opponents
	Analyse their arguments
	Develop counter arguments
Advance the policy	Convince audiences that a given policy or action is the best solution for addressing the health issue
Intermediate	
Initiate and sustain influence on the policy-making process	Make it clear what action audiences can take to show their support
	Reinforce the political pressure exerted via lobbying and community action
Long term	
Policy change	

1. What is the problem?
   Gather key facts about the specific issue, its prevalence, which population groups are affected, and determinants of the problem (underlying causes). Although the causes of the problem will be complex, try to develop a concise statement of the problem focused on one specific aspect that the advocacy campaign is seeking to influence.
2. What is the solution?
   Specify a clear 'public health' policy solution. Present evidence to argue why it is likely to be effective. Locate existing success stories. If evidence is not available, present this in terms of a 'call for more research' to investigate if this solution will work. Are there small, strategic goals that could be achieved as an interim step towards more long-term change? The Health Communication Unit (2000) recommends structuring this around the following questions:
   o   What health issues are related to the policy?
   o   What are the financial and health costs of the related health issues?
   o   What will the costs of adopting or not adopting the policy be?

o   What valid and convincing evidence is there that a change in policy
     will have the desired effect – or that it is the most effective solution to
     achieve the public health goal?
3.   Who has the power to make the necessary change?
     This is the campaign's primary audience – those with decision-making
     power. Attribute responsibility to the individuals, organisations or gov-
     ernment body that has the decision-making power to change policy.
     Personalise the issue and identify key decision-makers by name. Frame
     their decision-making role in terms of wider social responsibility, public
     interest values and ethical issues.
4.   Who must be mobilised to apply the pressure for change?
     These are the campaign's secondary audiences – those with the power to
     influence decision-makers. Consider which groups in the public sector, pri-
     vate sector and community are likely to have the most influence and what
     are the best options for communicating with them? Which groups have
     already gained traction on this issue and are there ways to collaborate
     with them? What approaches can be used to engage other people who are
     stakeholders in the issue?
5.   What message would convince those with power to act for change?
     Consider, what is already known about each audience and what informa-
     tion is still needed? The message will need to be adapted for each audience
     group depending on their values, political ideologies and organisational
     goals. Wallack et al. (1999: 13) recommend that a compelling and
     persuasive message should be framed to appeal to the 'head, heart, hand
     and pocket-book'.
     Within this schema, head refers to the use of rational argument backed by
     compelling evidence. Heart involves appealing to commonly shared pub-
     lic values, such as fairness; freedom; social justice; family; environmental
     sustainability; ethical and emotional issues such as protection of children,
     family, human rights, vulnerability, abuse of power, deceitful or dishon-
     est behaviour. Hand frames the issue in terms of positive relationships,
     strong communities and a cohesive society. It clarifies what communities
     stand to lose if the policy is *not* adopted. Lastly, pocket book frames the
     policy solution in terms of financial good sense and responsible economic
     management in which the benefits outweigh the costs.

Identifying the campaign message

The campaign will require a key message that is brief, clear and consistent
across all media and all communication strategies. This is often modified over
time as small wins are achieved and new targets for change are established. Any
facts and figures should be presented using language and graphics that are easily understood by journalists and the public. Chapman (2007) recommends the
use of 'creative epidemiology' to express epidemiological data in more meaningful and powerful ways. For example, local relevance can be emphasised
whereby, instead of reporting 18,000 deaths per year, advocates talk in terms
of 10 deaths each day in their own city. Comparative statements can also be

useful, such as, 'more UK women die from breast cancer each month than have died from AIDS in the past decade'.

Finally, Ricketts (2012) suggests it is better to focus on one issue at a time, rather than multiple aspects of a complex problem. As we noted earlier in this chapter, all communications should carry a simple message that clearly states the problem, the solution, the power-holders and the actions people can take to get involved in generating change.

Designing the media strategy

It is essential to develop a 'media strategy' plan. According to Mindframe Media (2011), most important first step, and one that is frequently overlooked by inexperienced advocacy practitioners, is to be clear about the media policy of the group or organisation. This helps to establish how the group will work with the media (proactive or responsive) and what issues their spokespersons will/will not discuss. At this point, procedures should be established to outline what actions individuals should take when approached by the media and clear protocols about how media requests will be managed. In the following section, we outline key elements of the media strategy plan, tips for contacting the media and responding to requests, and we provide an overview of commonly used advocacy tools.

Media strategy plan
Identify audiences and the key message. Ensure that the primary and secondary audience(s) are identified (see the above section, 'Target audiences for Advocacy'). Make a clear statement of the key campaign message(s). Document the advocacy group's position on key related issues.

Select media channels and methods. Identify which media are accessed by each audience. Select the channels and methods that will reach the target audience. Media channels may include a mix of print, TV, radio and online media, while common 'methods' include news, current affairs, features and talkshows. Investigate which options for utilising social media are likely to (i) engage target audiences and (ii) assist the campaign in achieving its objectives (see Chapter 9).

Identify appropriate spokespeople. Mindframe Media (2011) emphasise the importance of engaging patients, consumers, carers and others with real-life experience of the issue as campaign spokespersons. As we noted in Chapter 6, people's participation in the process of telling their personal stories, through their own media-making on video, recorded interviews, photographs and/or speaking in public, can be deeply empowering for. However, advocacy groups need to ensure that all spokespersons are supported throughout the process of engaging with the media, so they feel well prepared and in a better position to maintain control over how their work is used and how they are represented (see Chapter 9). According to Chapman (2007), it is also essential to engage an expert as a spokesperson for the campaign, in order to bring an important human dimension to statistics and research reports. Ask them to provide a clear, concise and accessible short list of key facts. Prepare a ten second 'grab' with the main message. Keep in mind that for radio, 'soundbites' from an expert are usually less than seven seconds (Chapman et al. 2009).

Contacting the media
Prepare and send out a *media release* (see e.g. Figure 10.4) to each selected media outlet, with the appropriate news angle and language likely to appeal to their target audience. This is usually accompanied by a *background brief* containing important facts, figures and expert sources of further information. Digital files, such as photographs, or links to short soundbites and video clips designed as ready-to-use materials for journalists, can be supplied with the media release. It is important to remember that the media release is not itself a news story. The function of the media release is to attract the journalist's attention to a potential story, include key messages and provide further resources and spokespersons they can use as the raw materials for constructing their story.

A *media alert* is often used to inform the media about a newsworthy activity, such as a community event, stakeholder forum, press conference, including the time, date and location, so that they can send a journalist to cover the story. Follow up with a phone call and/or email to offer further assistance. For established media contacts, a phone call or brief email can be enough to prompt a story. Practical tips for writing media releases, a background brief and alerts can be found in Chapman (2007) and PHAIWA (2013a).

Responding to media requests
Mindframe Media (2011) emphasises the importance of planning ahead. Prepare a brief checklist of three main points and the campaign's main message. These should be short, pithy statements that the spokesperson can get across even if the interviewer doesn't ask for them. Make a short list of key facts or evidence. This gives the spokesperson authority and positions them as the expert. Anticipate the difficult questions an interviewer might ask.

Tools for media advocacy

As we discussed earlier in this chapter, the media release is one of the most common tools for media advocacy. We have provided an example of media release in Figure 10.4, along with a selection of practical formatting and content tips drawn from Mindframe Media (2011). The original media release, titled 'Nursing Homes "Bad Option" for Young People', was developed by Summer Foundation. Interested readers can access several examples of the associated media coverage, including a radio interview (ABC Radio National 2012), online news article (Winkler and Callaway 2012) and a rural community newspaper article (Knight 2012).

SUMMER
FOUNDATION

Date for release

Organisation logo

Media release
Embargoed until 8 am Mon 9 July 2012

Short, clear, attention grabbing title

Nursing homes 'bad option' for young people

Research published today provides further evidence that young people should not be forced to live in nursing homes because there is nowhere else for them

First sentence is high impact. Main message

Simple language. Avoid jargon.

The Summer Foundation and Monash University conducted interviews with 68 people with disabilities and families who received services through the five-year Victorian Younger People in Residential Aged Care (YPIRAC) initiative. Summer Foundation CEO Dr Di Winkler said, 'This study shows that moving out of nursing homes enriches the lives of young people with disability. They go outside more often, have more opportunities to make everyday choices, have greater social interaction and spend fewer hours in bed.'

Summarise important points: who, what, where, when, how and why?

Human interest: personal story. Quote

Said Nicole, aged 33, 'When I was told I had the opportunity to move out of a nursing home I couldn't wait... It was great to get out. Now I am in my new home with other young people. I can talk. I can go to bed when I want. I can eat when I want to. I have got my own space... If I want to go outside I can go out now. It's so different here to the nursing home – I wanted to get out. I couldn't, I was locked in...The doors were locked.'

Compelling facts and statistics

Quote from expert sources

In 2006 the federal, state and territory governments funded a $244 million National YPIRAC program that ended in 2011. At the start there were 1,014 people aged under 50 in nursing homes, and there were still 621 in nursing homes in May 2011. 'Whilst this program has made a tremendous difference to the lives of people who received funding to either stop them going into a nursing home or moved them out, there are no new packages available to prevent new admissions of young people to nursing homes,' said Di Winkler.

'Although it is expected the National Disability Insurance Scheme (NDIS) will provide the funding for the support this target group needs to be able to live in the community, it will not address the chronic shortage of housing options for young people in nursing homes,' said Dr Winkler, 'More housing services must be built and Australia needs services that prevent nursing home admissions and create pathways back to community living, such as slow stream rehabilitation. If the Government does not change the system, 200 people under 50 will still be admitted to nursing homes each year in Australia.'

Restate the problem and policy solution

Contact person details incl. out of hours. 'Talent' for interview

'Nursing homes have an important function in our society,' said Disability Discrimination Commissioner Graeme Innes, 'But they are no place for young people with disability.'

(ends)

Pithy, memorable closing statement

Further Information: You can watch Nicole's digital story at http://youtu.be/3dZ_V4jvB1E To arrange an interview with a family member of a young person in a nursing home or for further comment, contact Carolyn Finis at Summer Foundation Ltd on 03 9894 7006 or 0431 311 969

Link to video.

Source of facts and statistics

Citation Guide: Winkler, D., Holgate, N., Sloan, S. & Callaway, L. (2012). *Evaluation of Quality of Life Outcomes of the Younger People in Residential Aged Care Initiative in Victoria*. Melbourne: Summer Foundation Ltd.

Organisation profile

About the Summer Foundation: The Summer Foundation is developing an integrated housing model for young people with disability that has the potential to resolve the issue of young people in nursing homes in Australia.

Summer Foundation Ltd. ABN 901 17 516 528 PO Box 208 Blackburn VIC 3130
Tel) 03 9894 7006 Fax) 03 8456 6325 http://www.summerfoundation.org.au

Organisation letterhead and contact details

Figure 10.4   Example media release

Other advocacy tools include:

- interviews (radio or television);
- radio grab;
- letter to the editor;
- feature story;
- website;
- digital advocacy tools, including SMS, social media and dedicated activist networking tools, online polling, petitions, action alerts and direct email lobbying.

Tools for digital, or e-advocacy, using email, petitions and social media are covered in Chapter 9. We also recommend readers spend time exploring the websites of the advocacy organisations in chapters 9 and 10 to become familiar with how this works in practice. Excellent practical guides are available to assist organisations in developing and using the above tools for their own advocacy work (see PHAIWA 2013a; Shaw 2013; Ricketts 2012; Mindframe Media 2011; Chapman 2007).

Other useful public health advocacy websites include:

- Australian Health Promotion Association – http://www.healthpromotion. org.au/advocacy
  This organisation provides advocacy information and resources including journal articles, guides, tool kits and websites to enable health promotion practitioners to engage in effective action at the national, branch and local levels. Excellent examples of resources include submissions to politicians and members of government, responses received, position papers, media releases and letters.
- ASH Scotland – http://www.ashscotland.org.uk/media.aspx
  Press releases, media facts, organisational profile, personal stories, evidence base, presentations, evidence and persuasive 'at-a-glance' statistics.
- Tobacco Free Kids – http://global.tobaccofreekids.org/en/
  Advocacy case studies, fact sheets, media releases, presentations, practical toolkits and manuals.

CHAPTER SUMMARY

- Public health advocacy aims to create social, physical and legislative environments that make it easier for people to be healthy. It involves practitioners and community members working together for change.
- Public health advocacy seeks policy changes that support the development of health promoting environments – in local communities and wider society. It involves strategic communication to shape public opinion, mobilise the community and influence decision-makers.

cont.

- Key strategies include media advocacy, political lobbying and community action. Media advocacy works with the media to set the agenda, shape public debates, discredit the opposition and advance policy development. Political lobbying uses more direct communication with policy-makers, politicians and government to influence decision-making. Community action maintains public pressure on decision-makers through coalitions and alliances involving community groups and professionals.

- Public health advocacy is a contentious process that is often conducted in the face of opposition from powerful and highly organised politicians, industry and vested interest groups.

- Advocacy groups need to make strategic use of the media to influence news coverage, public discussion and political debate between supporters and opponents of change.

- Effective advocacy relies on constructing clear and convincing arguments for policy change that combine compelling evidence with creative rhetorical strategies. These arguments can be used to raise awareness of a health problem, describe the causes, outline effective policy solutions and identify who is responsible for creating change.

- Public health professionals and health practitioners are in an ideal position to influence policy decision-makers by drawing attention to the health implications of their policies. We can influence policy directly, through becoming involved in the policy-making process, or indirectly by voting in elections and/or joining an advocacy group seeking to influence decision-makers in governments and corporations. As health professionals, we also have a responsibility to be proactive in raising awareness amongst our colleagues and communities about ways health is influenced by economic and other policy decisions. This includes encouraging others to become political advocates for the changes needed to improve public health and to make the most of every opportunity to influence these decisions.

References

Action on Smoking and Health 2013. Accessed 6 May 2014 http://ash.org.

ABC Radio National 2012, 'Australia lacking age appropriate residential care', *RN Drive*, 9 July 2012. Accessed 6 May 2014 http://www.abc.net.au/radionational/programs/drive/australia-lacking-age-appropriate-residential-care/4119524.

ASH Scotland 2013. Accessed 6 May 2014 www.ashscotland.org.uk.

Baum, F. 2008, *The New Public Health: An Australian Perspective*, Third Edition, Oxford, Melbourne.

Brown, P., Zavestoski, S., McCormick, S., Mayer, B., Morello-Frosch, R. and Gasior Altman, R. 2004a, 'Embodied health movements: New approaches to social movements in health', *Sociology of Health and Illness*, 26 (1): 50–80.

Chapman, S. 1994, 'What is public health advocacy?', in S. Chapman and D. Lupton (eds), *The Fight for Public Health*, BMJ Publishing Group, London, 3–12.

Chapman, S. 2004, 'Advocacy for public health: A primer', *Journal Epidemiology and Community Health*, 58: 361–365.

Chapman, S. 2007, *Public Health Advocacy and Tobacco Control: Making Smoking History*, Blackwell, Oxford.

Chapman, S. Holding, S., Ellerm, J., Heenan, R., Fogarty, A., Imison, M., Mackenzie, R. and McGeechan, K. 2009, 'The content and structure of Australian television reportage on health and medicine, 2005–2009: Parameters to guide health workers', *Medical Journal of Australia*, 191: 620–624.

Chapman, S. 2013, *Over Our Dead Bodies: Port Arthur and Australia's Fight for Gun Control*, Sydney University Press, Sydney.

Chappell, B. 2012, 'Canada stops its defense of asbestos, as Quebec's mines close for good', *NPR*, 17 September 2012. Accessed 6 May 2014 http://www.npr.org/blogs/thetwo-way/2012/09/17/161298741/canada-stops-its-defense-of-asbestos-quebecs-mines-shut-down.

Dreher, T. 2010, 'Cultural diversity and the media', in S. Cunningham and G. Turner (eds), *The Media and Communications in Australia*, Allen & Unwin, Crows Nest, 273–284.

Every Australian Counts 2013, 'Coalition sticks with NDIS and unveils disability policy', *News*, 20 August 2013. Accessed 6 May 2014 http://everyaustraliancounts.com.au/category/news/.

Freudenberg, N., Bradley, S. and Serrano, M. 2009, 'Public health campaigns to change industry practices that damage health: An analysis of 12 case studies', *Health Education and Behaviour*, 36 (2): 230–249 (April 2009). doi: 10.1177/1090198107301330.

Gould, T., Fleming, M. and Parker, E. 2012, 'Advocacy for health: Revisiting the role of health promotion', *Health Promotion Journal of Australia*, 23 (3): 165–170.

Green, J. and Tones, K. 2010, *Health Promotion Planning and Strategies and Methods*, 2nd Edition, Sage, London.

Johnson, S. 2009, *Public Health Advocacy. Healthy Public Policy Discussion Paper*. Alberta Health Services: Edmonton, Alberta.

Keleher, H. and C MacDougall, C, 2011, *Understanding Health*, Third Edition, Oxford, Melbourne.

Knight, H. 2012, 'Improved care urged for young people', *Bendigo Advertiser*, 9 July 2012. Accessed 6 May 2014 http://www.bendigoadvertiser.com.au/story/138904/improved-care-urged-for-young-people/.

Labonte 1994 in Gould, T., Fleming, M. L. and Parker, E. 2012, 'Advocacy for health: Revisiting the role of health promotion', *Health Promotion Journal of Australia*, 23 (3): 165–170.

Laverack, G. 2013, *Health Activism: Foundations and Strategies*, Sage, London.

Mindframe Media 2011, *Suicide and Mental Illness in the Media. A Mindframe Resource for the Mental Health and Suicide Prevention Sectors*, Commonwealth of Australia, Canberra.

Orlowski, J. 1989, 'It's time for pediatricians to "rally round the pool fence"', *Pediatrics*, 83 (6): 1065–1066.

Parents Jury 2013. Accessed 6 May 2014 www.parentsjury.org.au.

Parvanta, C., Nelson, D., Parvanta, S. and Harner, R. 2011, *Essentials of Public Health Communication*, Jones and Bartlett Learning, Sudbury, MA.

Peacock, M. 2009, *Killer Company*, ABC Books, Melbourne.

Peacock, M. 2011, *Toxic Trade*, Foreign Correspondent, Australian Broadcasting Corporation, http://www.abc.net.au/foreign/video_archive_2011.htm 8/11/2011. Video avail on 'Flash' but access to transcript has ended, http://www.abc.net.au/foreign/content/2011/s3359246.htm.

Public Health Advocacy Institute of Western Australia 2013a, *Public Health Advocacy Toolkit*, 3rd Edition, Curtin University, Perth. Accessed 6 May 2014 www.phaiwa. org.au.

Public Health Advocacy Institute of Western Australia 2013b, *What Is Public Health Advocacy?* Accessed 6 May 2014 http://www.phaiwa.org.au/fact-sheets/258-advocacy-factsheet.

Reber, B. and Kim, J. 2006, 'How activist groups use websites in media relations: Evaluating online press rooms', *Journal of Public Relations Research*, 18: 2, 313–333.

Ricketts, A. 2012, *The Activists Handbook: A Step-By-Step Guide to Participatory Democracy*, Zed Books, London.

Shaw, R. 2013, *The Activist's Handbook: Winning Social Change in the 21st Century*, 2nd Edition, University of California Press, Berkeley.

Singhal, A. 2011, 'Juanita publicly asks "What will you do for me, mayoral candidate?" Children, media and health advocacy in Colombia', in C. Von Feilitzen, U. Carlsson and C. Bucht (eds), *Yearbook 2011: News Questions, New Insights, New Approaches,* Nordicom International Clearing House on Children, Youth and Media, Gothenburg, 145–156.

Summer Foundation 2012, *Annual Report 2012*. Summer Foundation, Melbourne.

Summer Foundation 2013, *Annual Report 2013*. Summer Foundation, Melbourne.

Talbot, L. and Verrinder, G. 2005, 'Working for change: Healthy public policy to create supportive environments', *Promoting Health: The Primary Health Care Approach*, Elsevier, Sydney, 77–91.

Talbot, L. and Verrinder, G. 2014, *Promoting Health: A Primary Health Care Approach*, Elsevier, Sydney.

The Health Communication Unit (THCU) 2000, *Media Advocacy Workbook*, Centre for Health Promotion, University of Toronto, Ontario, Canada.

Waldman, S. 2011, *The Information Needs of Communities: The Changing Media Landscape in a Broadband Age*, US Federal Communications Commission, Washington, DC.

Wallack, L., Woodruff, K., Dorfman, L. and Diaz, I. 1999, *News for a Change: An Advocate's Guide to Working with the Media*, Sage, Thousand Oaks.

Winkler, D. and Callaway, L. 2012, 'Young people in nursing homes denied basic human rights', *The Conversation*, 12 July 2012. Accessed 6 May 2014 http://theconversation.com/young-people-in-nursing-homes-denied-basic-human-rights-8176.

WHO 1998, *Health Promotion Glossary* [Internet]. Geneva (CHE). WHO 1998. Accessed 6 May 2014 http://www.who.int/healthpromotion/about/HPR%20Glossary%201998.pdf.

WHO 2005, 'Proceedings of the 6th Global Conference on Health Promotion [Internet]', August 2011. Bangkok, Thailand, 2005. Available from http://www.lydheilsustod.is/media/lydheilsa/bankok_charter_healthprom_gloablisedw.pdf.

WHO 2012, '2012: Tobacco interference'. Accessed 6 May 2014 http://www.euro.who.int/en/health-topics/disease-prevention/tobacco/world-no-tobacco-day/2012-tobacco-industry-interference.

Index

LIBRARY, UNIVERSITY OF CHESTER